Reiki for Beginners

Self Healing Mindfulness Meditation Guide for Your Aura Cleansing, Increase and Balance Your Life Energy

(Developing Your Abilities for Energy)

Frank De Dan

Published by Rob Miles

Frank De Dan

All Rights Reserved

Reiki for Beginners: Self Healing Mindfulness Meditation Guide for Your Aura Cleansing, Increase and Balance Your Life Energy (Developing Your Abilities for Energy)

ISBN 978-1-989990-31-5

All rights reserved. No part of this guide may be reproduced in any form without permission in writing from the publisher except in the case of brief quotations embodied in critical articles or reviews.

Legal & Disclaimer

The information contained in this book is not designed to replace or take the place of any form of medicine or professional medical advice. The information in this book has been provided for educational and entertainment purposes only.

The information contained in this book has been compiled from sources deemed reliable, and it is accurate to the best of the Author's knowledge; however, the Author cannot guarantee its accuracy and validity and cannot be held liable for any errors or omissions. Changes are periodically made to this book. You must consult your doctor or get professional medical advice before using any of the suggested remedies, techniques, or information in this book.

Upon using the information contained in this book, you agree to hold harmless the Author from and against any damages, costs, and expenses, including any legal fees potentially resulting from the application of any of the information provided by this guide. This disclaimer applies to any damages or injury caused by the use and application, whether directly or indirectly, of any advice or information presented, whether for breach of contract, tort, negligence, personal injury, criminal intent, or under any other cause of action.

You agree to accept all risks of using the information presented inside this book. You need to consult a professional medical practitioner in order to ensure you are both able and healthy enough to participate in this program.

Table of Contents

INTRODUCTION 1

CHAPTER 1: REIKI MEDITATION 4

CHAPTER 2: TIPS TO INCREASE YOUR ENERGY WITH REIKI 20

CHAPTER 3: WHAT TO KNOW BEFORE UNDERGOING REIKI TREATMENT 27

CHAPTER 4: SELF-CONSCIOUSNESS 31

CHAPTER 5: WHAT ARE THE BENEFITS AND LIMITS OF REIKI? 53

CHAPTER 6: THE THIRD EYE; BACKGROUND AND HISTORY 66

CHAPTER 7: THE BENEFITS OF REIKI HEALING 76

CHAPTER 8: HISTORY OF REIKI 80

CHAPTER 9: THE DEFINITION OF REIKI: 87

CHAPTER 10: PRINCIPLES OF REIKI 108

CHAPTER 11: BODY, DISEASE AND EMOTIONAL ISSUES 129

CHAPTER 12: REIKI FOR SELF-HEALING 148

CHAPTER 13: HOW REIKI INCREASE YOUR ENERGY, REDUCE STRESS, DEPRESSION AND IMPROVE YOUR HEALTH 168

CHAPTER 14: POSITIONS FOR THE APPLICATION 174

CONCLUSION 183

Introduction

Hello there, come in, come in, don't be shy – welcome, welcome.

First of all, allow us to thank you for buying this little book.

If you're feeling a little mixed in your emotions right now, don't worry, it's quite all right, in fact it's quite understandable.

On the one hand you may be feeling somewhat nervous and excited, hoping beyond hope this book lives up to all your expectations.

On the other you may be feeling a little fearful in case it doesn't.

And there in the background may be lurking a little disappointment, because, after the excitement of building yourself up to buying the book – it's now actually arrived on your computer and its very arrival may have begun to burst those delicate bubbles of expectation and hope.

We do understand these feelings, as we've already said, but please be assured; we'll do our very best not to let you down.

Our aim is to help you discover the wonders of Reiki for yourself, and also to give you the tiniest glimpse into the world of metaphysics.

We want to help you see, maybe for the first time, the glorious you that you truly are...

Strong, powerful, beautiful, unstoppable and...

...most importantly - divine.

You are about to embark on a journey of discovery.

A journey of self-discovery, to be more precise, which can lead you to a place of contentment, meaning, fulfilment, happiness and joy.

Notice we have said a journey of discovery – not a journey of learning.

There is nothing in life you have to learn.

Let us repeat that for more emphasis.

There is nothing in life you have to learn.

You already know all there is to know.

This book has been written to gently remind you of this knowledge and help bring it more fully into your waking consciousness.

It is, therefore, a process of rediscovering that which you already know to be true.

It's about remembering who you are and why you are here.

You see, you are an incredibly powerful spiritual being; only you have chosen to forget all about it.

You have chosen to experience temporary spiritual amnesia.

We're going to act as the catalyst to help you restore your memory and return you to your senses.

Through reading these pages it's our wish that you become more fully aware of the incredible power you hold within yourself.

Chapter 1: Reiki Meditation

Meditation may seem very complicated or difficult to do, which pushes people away from ever giving it a try. In reality, it is actually one of the easiest things to begin doing, although true greatness comes with practice and patience. At its core, meditation is simply a process in which you sit with yourself and use various techniques and tools to focus the mind and bring about a sense of calm and peace.

Through sitting with yourself, often in silence, you allow yourself a moment to disconnect from the hectic world around you and to really focus on your own thoughts and feelings. You can see what is stressing you out, what is hurting, what emotions you are overwhelmed by, and what persistent thoughts are attacking your mind. As you allow all of this to flow in, you acknowledge that it exists, and then you simply let it go from your mind, body, and soul.

Learning how to meditate is easy and accessible to anyone who would like to try it, although being able to engage in it for long periods of time does take practice. We are so used to our minds constantly being stimulated and engaged that it can be difficult to motivate ourselves to simply sit and exist.

Why is Meditation Fundamental to Reiki?

Meditation is a core aspect of Reiki because it allows both the practitioner and the client to get in touch with their own energy and experience. Most Reiki practitioners will engage in a quick form of meditation prior to beginning any session, and they will also often use meditation in their own day to day life. Meditation allows us to connect with ourselves, but it also welcomes divine energy into us. It can allow us to understand a higher truth, but it can also calm our minds and prepare them for any healing that is about to come our way.

Meditation is all about transformation, and it is through the process of meditating that we participate in transforming our own lives and our own experiences. We begin to have a grasp on our minds, and instead of being controlled by our thoughts, we learn to control them. You can learn how to replace anger with compassion, sadness with gratefulness, and anxiety with excitement. You will energize yourself, learn to truly love yourself, and ultimately be comfortable within your own truth.

When you pair these benefits with Reiki, you are given a practitioner who is more attune and more aware. They not only understand the divine energy, but they also understand their own energy and how it functions in their own bodies. They can make the practitioner more at peace and clear their mind of their own problems before they work with a client. By purifying themselves through meditation, Reiki healers can offer more pure healing, as there is no risk of transferring their own negative energy onto someone else.

Even if you are not a practitioner, meditation can be used in conjunction with your Reiki treatments in order to continue the benefits that were seen in the session. Reiki can help heal you at the moment, but it is up to you to maintain that, and through meditation, you can tap into that healing energy and feel it working inside of you.

If your mind is constantly talking to you, give it a break, and try meditation. Learn to thrive inside the silence, and welcome the break from the fast-paced world that we live in. The only true way to achieve ultimate inner peace is by incorporating meditation into your everyday routine. You will gain real control over your mind and thoughts, experience a deeper calmness and mental clarity, and be more in touch with the spiritual energy that runs throughout you.

And meditation is not simply a spiritual technique, but rather something that is backed and endorsed by science and medical professionals. Constant stress is very harmful to us, and if we don't find ways to cope with and master that stress, then we can end up sick or worse. Meditation is great for removing that stress from our lives, as well as teaching us better coping strategies and making us realize that we don't have to succumb to the stress but rather that we can transform it into something positive.

When Dr. Mikao Usui came to understand Reiki, he learned that simply healing a person's energy wasn't enough to create long term change. Instead, after encountering individuals whose bodies he had healed and seeing they were still struggling, he understood that healing the mind was the second piece of the equation. This is why Reiki and meditation are so closely linked, for true healing only comes when all parts of us are at peace.

Learning How to Meditate

When you first start out learning to meditate, it is important that you are patient with yourself as well as the process. Most of us are not accustomed to sitting still in silence with nothing to distract us, and that is one of the many excuses people use as to why they cannot meditate. Some of the common excuses also include:

- I don't enough time to meditate
- Meditation won't work for me
- My brain refuses to shut off
- I'm uncomfortable with silence
- I get bored too easily
- I get too distracted by other things
- I can't stick with it
- I'm not doing it right
- I don't want to be alone with my thoughts

But in reality, none of these excuses are valid ones, because all of them can be combated through meditation. Let's break a few of the excuses and see why meditation is actually beneficial instead of something to be avoided.

"I Don't Have Enough Time to Meditate"

We all lead busy lives, where we most likely work or go to school as well as having family and household commitments on top of it. Adding in meditation may seem like an impossible task, as there simply isn't enough time in the day for everything. But meditation doesn't need to take long, as it can be done anywhere at any time. From quick 5 minute sessions, to longer 30 minute ones, these are all easy to fit into the day if you want to. Maybe you wake up 15 minutes earlier so you can meditate before your shower. Or maybe you take 15 minutes before bed to just sit quietly and practice. No matter when you choose to do it, it still leaves you 23 hours and 45 minutes each day for everything else.

"Meditation Won't Work for Me"

There isn't anyone on this planet that meditation doesn't work for, and that is because it isn't some crazy concept or spiritual activity that requires special education or a certain belief system. Instead, all it is is giving yourself a moment to relax and exist without having to do anything else. Even if all you do is sit quietly and breathe, you're automatically reducing your stress levels and calming your mind without any extra effort. By the time the 15 minutes are up, you will feel relaxed whether or not you want to.

"I Get Bored Too Easily"

This is actually a pretty valid excuse, but not in the sense that it should prevent you from meditating. In fact, if you get bored so easily that you cannot go 15 minutes without being distracted, then you could benefit from meditation even more so. With social media and television and all of the gadgets we interact with, there is almost no time in the day where our brains aren't stimulated and distracted.

But this prevents us from spending time alone with ourselves and getting to know our minds on a personal level. Instead of shying away from boredom, embrace it. After a while, you will come to love your personal, quiet time, and instead of being bored, you will simply be calm.

"I Don't Know How to Do It, and I Can't Do It Right"

There is no right or wrong way to meditate, only suggestions, guidance, and various techniques. When we break meditation down to its basics, we see that it simply, you spending time with you. You can do it sitting, standing, or lying down and you can do it for as little or as long as you like. You can play music in the background, follow a guided tutorial, or sit and think of nothing at all. You may think about various things, you make become distracted, you may feel bored, you may be completely absorbed in it, or you may just focus on your breathing. All of this is fine, normal, and part of the meditation process.

So, if we remove these excuses from our minds, what are we left with? How do we begin meditation, and how exactly do we learn to do it? Follow these steps in order to try meditation for the first time:

Find a time in the day where you can set aside five minutes without being interrupted

Go somewhere quiet where you won't be bothered by anyone, such as your bedroom

Sit comfortably, or lay down, and then set a five minute timer

Close your eyes and begin breathing normally

As you breathe, begin focusing on your breath and feel each inhale and exhale and how it affects the body

If you begin to think of something else, simply return your mind to your breath

When the timer goes off, you are done

And that is really all there is to it. This is meditation at its simplest form, and there is no need to get extravagant or make it into something more complicated than it actually is. As you get accustomed to doing five minutes a day, you can start to increase the time. Move to ten, fifteen, and even thirty minute sessions. So long as it is helping you, then you are doing it correctly.

Once you feel accomplished with the very basics of meditation, there are numerous variations that you can try in order to unlock different parts of your mind. Next, we will look at different meditations, how to do them, and what the benefits are of each.

Different Meditations to Try

We know that meditation can offer numerous health benefits, but did you know that there are different meditations depending on what you are trying to achieve? Some people go their entire lives only doing breath meditation, and if that works for them, then it is perfect. But others find that breath meditation doesn't go deep enough, or they enjoy variety, and so they seek out other techniques in order to satisfy these needs. Let's look at some of the various ways in which we can meditate in order to benefit our mind, body, and spirit.

Concentration Meditation

The basic meditation that we discussed earlier is a form of concentration meditation, but it is only one version of many. This technique is used to develop our concentration skills, and to give yourself a focal point in case you find yourself getting distracted during your practice. Instead of simply focusing on the breath, you can choose to focus on anything that you like. Maybe you play a mantra or music, maybe you light a candle and watch the flame, maybe you hold a crystal in your hand and focus on that, or maybe you identify one of the chakras and keep that in your mind's eye. Whatever it is you choose, make sure it has meaning to you and is the subject of that meditation. Don't pick a dirty sock on the floor, unless you are trying to manifest the willpower to keep your room clean. Meditation is always about intention, so find what you are attending to achieve, and every time your mind wanders, bring it back to that focal point.

Mindfulness Meditation

This type of meditation is quite different, as you no longer have a focal point, such as the breath. Before, when the mind would wander, you would bring it back to the center, but now we want to encourage the mind to wander. In mindfulness meditation, the point is to be mindful of our thoughts and feelings and to let them float across our minds. As each thought comes you will acknowledge it, and then let it drift past as a new thought or emotion fills you. The purpose of this is to begin to understand how we think and feel, and to detect the patterns in our own mind. There is no judgment on your part or even any involvement, you simply are observing how your mind works. Over time you will learn how you think, why you think that way, and be better equipped to handle your thoughts and take control of your mind.

Reiki Zen Meditation

Coming back to having a sort of focal point, this type of meditation is all about your Chi, or life energy. As you get into a meditative state, you want to seek out and find the energy that is flowing through your center. Once you are able to find and feel it, expand your experience, and notice how that energy pulsates out from the center and through your entire body. Trace the course of that energy as it moves from chakra to chakra, limb to limb, and simply allow it to envelop you. There is no need to use it as a focal point, but instead, simply acknowledge it and enjoy it.

The Center Finger Technique

Sometimes having a mental focal point isn't enough, and our minds will wander too far without us noticing and bringing them back to the center. Before you realize it, the timer is going off, and you have spent the last five minutes thinking all about what you are going to get to the grocery store later. To combat this, the center finger technique uses a physical feeling to pull your mind back and prevent it from wandering off. To do this, bring your fingertips together so that each one of the hands is touching its counterpart on the right hand. Now, focus completely on the middle fingers and the sensation of them pressing together. When your mind starts to wander, keep pressing the fingers together so that the physical pressure is enough to make your mind take notice.

Reiki Specific Meditation

During your Reiki education, you will be taught various forms of meditation that incorporate the healing hand movements with the focus of the mind. To practice these, however, you need to be taught by a Master so that they can show you the proper technique and so that they may attune you with the energy needed to conduct a session properly. Two of the most common Reiki specific meditations are:

- Joshin Kokyu Ho (Level 1)
- Hatsurei Ho (Level 2)

While you will not be able to learn these without taking the corresponding classes, you can incorporate some of the hand positions in your regular meditative practice. The most common hand position that people use is called "Gassho," and it simply involves bringing the hands into a prayer position and placing them against your chest. This helps to bring energy into your heart chakra, and also helps focus and calm the mind. Adding this to your meditation can connect you to a higher focus, create added stillness, and increase our intuitive nature.

These are only a handful of the various techniques that are available to you, and once you have mastered the basics, then it is encouraged that you explore all of the different options available. If you are having trouble getting started, then there are also plenty of guided meditations that you can use by playing while you meditate. Whatever feels best for you, is what you should do.

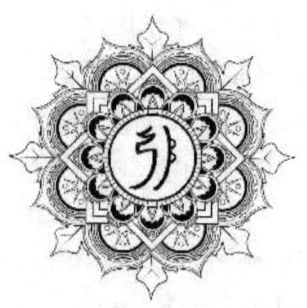

Chapter 2: Tips To Increase Your Energy With Reiki

The goal of Reiki is to make you feel better from the daily life anxieties. Here are some of the amazing lessons which will help you learn a lot through increasing the flow of Reiki by following on it accordingly. After getting done with the Reiki session, it is important that you follow these to keep the energy flow normal in the body.

1. Workout

Working out is necessary for everyone to stay active. It helps you keep the blood flowing normally and also keeps you away from catching a lot of diseases. People who start to work out in the young age, tend to stay healthier than anyone else throughout. Stretch, walk, jump or any sport you like but make sure you are in some kind of extra movement of the body to keep yourself going. It is like a self-treatment which you can do.

2. Shower well

Make sure to take a good detailed shower after the sessions you can take out all the toxins which are there externally. It is essential to keep yourself hygienic in order to stay away from the bacteria. You need to keep yourself clean to improve the hygiene. It will give you a good sleep and you will feel fresh after it. If you like to skip shower then do not skip it more than one day.

3. Work before eating

Do not consume food and then wait to workout. The best way for exercise to work on you is to do it empty stomach. Make sure that you do not fill yourself up but consider to do the workout in the morning when you wake up and then have juice after it. Then after a while you can have something to eat which will keep you fit all day long. Your metabolism gets strong when you work out daily and helps you to digest food quicker. It gives you all the possible nutrients which you need and takeout the wastes normally as well.

4. Get exposure

Make sure to sit under the sun once in a while to get the natural vitamin D. it is necessary along with the food that you take the extra sunlight from the back. Sit at a lawn and keep your back toward the sunlight so that you can get some warmth of it. It is essential for healthy skin and keeps you moisturized inside as well. It gives you energy and you will feel fresh after it for sure.

5. Stay warm

Make sure that you stay at a warm area during winters. Some people prefer to wear the layers of clothes during the winter season and think that they are protected. That is not the case, you need to stay at a warmer room where the atmosphere is warm as well. Keep yourself warm especially the feet and hand then you will see the entire body will respond normally and you will not feel extra cold as well.

6. Find shades

When you are exposed to the sunlight being outdoor, prefer to stay under a shade. Do not expose much to the sunlight directly because it can cause dehydration. Find a place to sit and keep yourself protected from the direct rays of sun for a long time for you.

7. Remind yourself

You will have to remind yourself that you have gone through the reiki sessions so that you can stay active. Make sure to wash your face and then repeat three times that you have had reiki sessions. It will activate the process in your mind and you will be able to feel the peace within yourself.

8. Visualize

Consider to do the visualization to feel better. Visualize your favorite color and then make something out it. Do not hold back from the imaginations because they can go far away and you won't regret it as well but enjoy it. Keep your eyes closed for a while and think of the most important things in your life and you will see the smile coming to your face all of a sudden.

9. Breathe slowly

Make sure to take out time and breathe slowly by inhaling and exhaling completely so that you can relax your body and think openly. You will see that your intuitions will work fast and you will experience a different side of life.

10. Play your favorite music

Music is extremely important for you to keep on going with a normal life. In the daily life, we tend to be so stressed that forget the fun of the life. So when you are going to get a reiki session, take along your favorite music and play it while you are getting the massage. You will feel how relaxing that will be and you will actually feel relieved of the stress from your brain and body. Check out the new albums and pick your favorites so you can get the best out of it.

11. Uncross the legs

You have to keep your legs straight or uncrossed when you are sitting. Crossed legs restrain your body to flow the blood normally in your body. You need to keep the movements going on and you also need to sit appropriately to make sure that the flow of blood keeps on going without any disturbances.

12. Stay patient

Make sure to be patient while you are getting the reiki session. You may not feel the outcome of it all of the sudden and some people may feel it suddenly so make sure to be patient with it. It will work eventually and you will feel lighter on your brain. The blood flowing starts after a while when the body warms up so be patient and have the courage to face it gently. You will see how happy your mood will be and when you start feeling that then you will realize that it is working now.

Chapter 3: What To Know Before Undergoing Reiki Treatment

Although research has been done on reiki's alleged healing benefits, none satisfy the strict criteria set by conventional scientific standards. You may have heard of various medical studies which prove reiki's efficacy—but that's simply hype at best, or mere wishful thinking.

It may surprise you to know that the American government has looked into alternative forms of medicine, and has spent about $2.5 billion dollars researching their efficacy over several decades. While some forms of alternative medicine have shown promising results (such as acupuncture), others like reiki have failed to pass muster—at least as of this writing (July 2015).

Nevertheless, it's hard to ignore the millions around the world who swear by reiki. On the understanding that science still doesn't have all the answers and that new discoveries are being made every day, it helps to keep an open mind.

The US Department of Health and Human Services has many sub-branches which look into and oversee many types of alternative medical treatments. One of these is the National Center for Complementary and Integrative Health (NCCIH). Although the NCCIH does not consider reiki to have any provable health benefits, it considers the practice to be safe and without any adverse side-effects, whatsoever. As such, it may be used together with conventional medical treatments. This is a very important point to consider.

If you do require treatment for something, please consult with your GP first. Reiki is harmless, but it should never be used as a stand-alone treatment for anything.

If you are a devout Roman Catholic, then you should know that the American Catholic Church does not recognize its validity. In 2009, the US Conference of Catholic Bishops came up with the "Guidelines for Evaluating Reiki as an Alternative Therapy." This document considers reiki to not only be bogus, it considers it to be incompatible with Catholic teaching. As such, its practice and promotion is forbidden in Catholic institutions, schools, and hospitals throughout the US, as well as by Catholic authorities and lay people.

Do note, however, that since the Vatican has not officially endorsed this document, Catholics of other countries are not obligated to observe the ruling. Further, we are not a theocracy here in America, so their ruling has no legal binding power. In fact, various American Catholics do practice reiki, as do a number of Catholic centers.

Whether or not reiki works for you, please use common sense. Do not ignore conventional medical treatment, or under any circumstances use reiki in lieu of it.

This book does not in any way endorse reiki as a valid form of medicine, nor does it make any claims regarding its efficacy. It only seeks to shed light on the practice and theory behind it.

Chapter 4: Self-Consciousness

What is self-consciousness? If we break it down on its phase value, it sounds harmless. After all, it is conscious of self, and it is something we need as human beings. In psychology, self-consciousness is an exaggerated attitude that we have on ourselves and how others perceive us. Self-consciousness is founded on wrong perceptions, and it can make us judge wrongly other's opinion. It changes behaviors that show our true selves and our natural interactions. Some of us are held back by self-consciousness.

Emotional Exploration

Our emotional world is formed from our feelings and life experiences. Our actions are a result of our feelings. When you combine these feelings with reasoning, they cause behaviors and actions of human beings. So, how should we explore these feelings? Let's look at the techniques to apply to understand how you feel the way you do. Focus on your breathing and settle your mind. Turn your attention to the emotion that is bothering your sadness, anger, or anxiety.

Listen to where you can feel it physically, arms, legs, or chest. To some people, it might be in different parts of the body; concentrate on the areas that the emotion is intense. Concentrate on the areas of discomfort.

You might experience discomfort or fear when you try to move closer to these feelings. It is okay; it is normal after all we have been running away from them for the better part of our lives. Be keen and don't try to liberate it. Try and tag your curiosity whiskers to this process.

Pay attention to the areas of discomfort and maintain your breath calmly. Close your eyes and imagine yourself sinking to the core of these feelings. At first, your mind will resist, but don't force it. Let it rest where it is, and after a minute, you can continue to imagine it sinking a little further. Repeat this 3 or 4 times until you feel like you are at the center of your heart's feelings.

At this last stage, let your body breathe in and out at the points of discomfort. Relax and keep your mind focused not to stray away from the points of discomfort. Rest at one point for several minutes and allow your awareness to widen.

This exercise should be done regularly, and by doing so, explore and understand your emotions well.

Emotional Consciousness

Self-conscious emotions are emotions like shame, guilt, pride, and embarrassment that help us to relate with our consciousness of how people react to us and our sense of self. We live in a social world, and other's people's perception of us is important to move to the next level. In schools we are examined by our teachers, in our careers, we are interviewed by the panel, and even in dates, the other party decides whether or not to be in a relationship with you. In today's world, social media and its pressures can increase our self-consciousness and anxiety. The current technological avenues like Facebook, Twitter, Instagram, and many others can facilitate self-consciousness, but those feelings have deeper roots.

Our inner voices and especially the critical voice, is deep-rooted in us from our childhood days to our adult phase. This negative voice can only be affected by our adult experiences but can never develop then. It comes from memories of the sufferings we experienced in our childhood. This trauma is not necessarily sexual abuse or physical abuse but even the small traumas that are experienced by children when growing up. We all experience such traumas in one way or another, and they are the cause of us feeling inferior or different from others.

We keep hearing this critical voice in our lives and the more we pay attention to it, the more conscious we feel. After understanding what self-consciousness is, let us now understand how it affects us.

When people feel like they have a negative attribute or even part of the body, they tend to change their behavior as a reaction to their self-consciousness. It can lead a person to lead a lonely life or to become a people-pleaser to be accepted. This feeling can stop us from interacting with others. Sometimes people equate self-consciousness to shyness as they feel embarrassed when doing some things or when interacting. These feelings can be mirrored in our body language and our facial expressions.

Our critical inner voice makes us more self-conscious, and when we listen to it, we may isolate ourselves and then judge ourselves harshly. We can only overcome self-consciousness by recognizing the destructive voices and work on countering them every day.

Emotional Mechanism

Emotion is the state of mind connected with the nervous system caused by chemical changes that are associated with feelings, thoughts, behavioral responses, and either pleasure or displeasure. The processing of emotional information and behavior is the role of the amygdala. Different studies have proven that plausible circuits transmit sensory inputs to amygdalae for the processing of emotions. What are the five basic emotions?

There are different types of emotions that influence how we live with each other. Sometimes, you might think that emotions rule us; choices, actions, and perceptions are influenced by emotions. The different types of emotions are:

· Happiness- We all strive to be happy in one way or another. Happiness is characterized by satisfaction, contentment, gratification, and well-being. We express this emotion through facial expressions, body language, and a lovely tone of voice.

· Sadness- Sadness is an emotion characterized by grief, disinterest, disappointment, and dampened the mood. We all experience this emotion from time to time, but to some people, it is prolonged and causes depression. How do we express this emotion? Through dampened mood, indolence, withdrawal, crying, or quietness.

· Fear- Fear keeps us away from dangerous situations and helps us to survive. Some people are sensitive to fear, and while some look for situations that provoke it. We express this emotion via our body language like opening our eyes wide, trying to run away from the threat, and awe experience a rapid heartbeat.

· Disgust- This is a sense of distaste. It can be expressed by different actions like vomiting, wrinkling our nose, and turning away from the disgusting object or smell.

· Anger- Anger is a good negative emotion. It can inspire you to act in case of something bothering you. How is it manifested? Throw frowning, turning away from your cause of anger, change of tone to yelling, sweating, hitting, throwing, and kicking objects.

· Surprise- It is a brief emotion that is negative, positive, or natural. This emotion is characterized by raising eyebrows, opening the mouth, jumping back, yelling or gasping. Studies surprising information stick to the memory longer.

· Other types of emotions- They are contentment, relief, shame, guilt, amusement, satisfaction, excitement, embarrassment, and pride in achievement.

The Deepness of Emotions

The deepness of emotions is how we experience and understand emotions.

How do we explore the deepness of our emotions?
- Intensity- We should feel the emotions with all intensity
- Feel the depth of the said emotions in our bodies.
- Depth of substance;
- Depth of space and time.

What are the characteristics of people who have discovered the deepness of emotions?
- They feel different emotions other than anger and happiness.
- They can accurately tell how they feel.
- They can differentiate their emotions. It means they know can tell what emotion they are feeling besides having over a hundred emotions in human beings.
- They can tell what caused their emotions and the reason.
- They are not ashamed to respond to their live events with their different feelings.

Deepness of emotions is not when emotions overcome people, and they have no idea of what is happening.

Mindfulness

It is a mental state of being aware of one's present moment. It can be realized through training, like meditation. People who live mindfully do not dwell on the past, and neither do they anticipate the future but live in the present. They internalize their thoughts and feelings and never judge them as wrong or right. Let us look at the benefits of mindfulness.

· People who practice mindfulness meditation have an increased working memory capacity.

· They can know their feeling and free their minds.

· They have lower anxiety levels and high self-esteem.

· They are focused and do not react easily with their emotions.

· They are attentive and concentrate more.

· They have low-stress levels.

· They can control physical pain.

Is mindfulness harmful? Everything with an advantage has a disadvantage, and mindfulness is no exception. Let us look at these disadvantages.

- People who practice mindfulness meditation are susceptible to false memories.

- In mindfulness meditation, people discard their negative thoughts to free their minds from negativity. This practice may make cause them to discard some positive thoughts which can be strengthening.

- Some people who practice mindfulness avoid strenuous tasks and prefer to stay in that state of mindfulness.

- It can cause some psychological and physical problems like hallucinations and derealization.

Know Yourself

Knowing yourself simply as it states understands your weaknesses and strengths, desire and dreams, passion, and fears. What are the benefits of knowing yourself?

· You will be happier with the ability to express your true self.

· You will have fewer internal conflicts because your actions will be in line with your feelings.

· Knowing yourself will help you make good decisions in life.

· You will have self-control.

· You will have the will-power to resist social pressures.

· When you know yourself, you become aware of your struggles, and that makes you empathetic. It enables you to understand and tolerate others.

· You become alive and excitingly experience life.

We should look at different ways to know ourselves, shouldn't we?

Know and understand your personality through reflection.

Know your core values by writing them down.

Learn and understand your body to set goals and know your limits.

Write a journal every day to reflect on yourself.

Recognize your weaknesses and strengths.

Have a mission and vision in life.

Cultural Exploration

We have different cultures in the world, and they play a great role in molding our self-consciousness. Our cultures were instilled in us from when we were young, and the roots are deep-rooted. Some people have explored different cultures, and this has opened their eyes more to how they view themselves. Some cultures can affect our self-consciousness negatively and other positives. In some cultures, women are taken and viewed as lesser human beings. They are denied a chance to give their opinion on matters that concern them and society. They have no right to express their feelings too. From their childhood to their adulthood, the society works on killing their self-consciousness and self-worth. It impacts a negative perception of themselves from a tender age while the men who dominate such cultures have inflated egos and acts like gods. We should strive to be aware of ourselves culturally; it is important, but we should not lose our self-worth because of some cultures we have no idea where they originated from. Being culturally aware is an act that starts with an individual before it drops to a group. Our cultures should unite us but not define us.

Highlighting Strengths

It is important to know our strengths to make the best out of ourselves. How do you identify your personal strengths? Your strengths are those things that are easier for you and probably giving other people some difficulties. You should utilize your strengths to the fullest because that is your competitive advantage. Knowing your strengths is like knowing the value that gives you self-awareness. When you know your strengths, you understand yourself better and how you function. Why should we focus on our strengths?

· It gives you increased positive emotions.

· Highlighting your strengths boosts your self-esteem.

· In capitalizing on our strengths, we become more successful.

Finding Blind Spots

Some of us never see the roles we play in making our problems. All of us have blind spots, and it is easier to spot them in others than in ourselves. Blind spots are weaknesses in us that hinder us from living our potential. It is easier to spot other people's blind spots than ours. Every one of us needs to see ourselves from other people's view. It is the beginning of self-consciousness. Finding blind spots is like placing cameras in our lives to watch how our actions contribute to troubles we would like to solve. It gives us a clear view of what is needed for our actions instead of blaming others.

Do you have blind spots? I know I said we all do, but are you aware of your blind spots? Finding your blind spots is a tough mission; it is an attack on your denial. Denial is worse than ignorance. It is the ability to make out the information and then not allowing it into our consciousness. Some information that is frightening or troubling gives us blind spots. It is a mind's way of protecting us. Identifying your blind spots is like going after the wind. Can you catch it? Well, it is tricky, but the good thing is that blind spots leave tracks. These tracks are repetitive life experiences that you can't explain. Some few examples are:
- You always find yourself in similar relationships despite the partners being different.
- Your fate never changes.
- People are always describing you in a way that you are not.
How do you get rid of your blind spots?

If you find tracks of repetitive experiences in your life, then you have blind spots. The easiest way to get rid of them is by being mindful. You should not be hard on yourself. Be patient with yourself and accept more consciousness. You should ask yourself the following questions to find help

- What am I scared to know?
- What is it that I am finding difficult to accept?
- What do I sense unknowingly?

Whatever answers that come to your mind are a sign of a big step towards self-consciousness, continue being patient and kind to yourself for big breakthroughs. These efforts are helpful for your self-awareness, but the better solution is asking for feedback from your friends and relatives. Honest feedback is valuable, and it can save you a lot of time.

Feedback

Feedback is important for a change and growth; what matters is how you handle it. Some feedbacks can break you or make you. We all hate receiving negative feedback, and we all react differently to them. Our reactions can be bad or right, but most of us are usually wrong.

Constructive feedback is formed on observations. It is focused on an issue and is specific. Here are the four types of feedback.

· Positive - It verifies annotations on past behavior. It focuses on successful behavior that we should continue with.

· Negative feedback- Corrects annotations about behaviors from the past. It looks at the unsuccessful behavior that should be rectified and never repeated.

· Negative feed-forward- Corrects annotations about behaviors in the future. It looks at the behavior that we should avoid in the future.

· Positive feed-forward- Verifies remarks about future behavior. It focuses on behavior that will enhance future performances.

When we receive feedback from friends and family, it is scary for all of us. Tough feedbacks are hard to digest, and most of us would rather run and hide than handle them. Tough feedbacks make us uncomfortable, and it hurts some people's esteem. How do you handle tough feedback? Use the below tactics to handle it like the expert you are.

Look for the positivity in it

Even in the harshest criticism, there is some positive information in it. Look for it and use it to build your self-consciousness. In such situations where you are the topic of criticism, your emotions might blind you from looking at the bigger picture. Nonetheless, you can ask a trusted friend or family member if there was any truth in the criticism. If their answer is yes, work on a change for a better tomorrow.

Look the bigger picture; the truth

Most of us view criticism negatively because we internalize as an attack on us. It is far from the truth. In fact, feedback is never about you, but your performance. We should avoid internalizing feedback not to hurt our esteem but instead listen to it and find the truth in it.

Think about the source

Before a reaction to any feedback, it is good to look at the source. Is it a person with the right information on the matter at hand and what the person's intentions are.

Walk away

In some cases, not all criticism is meant for our good. Some people are naturally mean. If the feedback is just some negative remarks meant to hurt you, take a step or two back for at least two minutes. No, I am not telling you to hide; this is meant to help you think clearly and not act on your emotions. Getting angry will not help you. You should end the situation with honesty and calmness.

Never forget that mean words target you for a negative reaction.

Move on

Apologize, correct your mistake, and move on.

Get curious

Never get on the defensive because of negative feedback but instead find out why through honest communication with the other person.

Put yourself in their shoes

Walk in the other person's shoes and try to understand them. Look at things from their end and see if they aimed to help or hurt you. With that in mind, it is a guarantee that you will have a good idea of the best response.

We can never avoid negative feedback, but we can teach ourselves how to deal with it. Any feedback is important as it helps us to grow and become self-conscious. Finally, remember we are in this together. Most of us have been there, too.

Chapter 5: What Are The Benefits And Limits Of Reiki?

Reiki helps to strengthen, realign, and recharge the life force within an individual. Below is a list of some of the major advantages that Reiki brings to its practitioners:
- Pain-free lifestyle
- Increased mobility, and less risk of arthritic ailments
- Reduction, and even eradication, of stress and anxiety
- Stabilized heart rate
- Healthy blood pressure levels
- Increased levels of immunity to illnesses
- Helps with dealing with the harsh side effects of chemotherapy
- Improves emotional well-being
- Positive outlook
- Enhances vitality exponentially
- Restores balance to our energy centers (chakras)

- Healthy levels of energy flowing to all organs, muscles, nerves, and bones
- Reduced fatigue
- Decreased likelihood of insomnia
- Increased ability to deal with change
- Assists in alcohol/addiction recovery
- Increased focus
- Calmness when dealing with otherwise stressful situations

There are almost limitless benefits that Reiki can offer.

However, it is important to note that Reiki is not a substitute for modern medicine. Nor is it a healing system that is at odds with modern medicine.

All of us can benefit from Reiki – our children, our parents and grandparents, and our animal companions.

Reiki for All Life Stages

Whatever an individual's need, Reiki normally can provide an adaptable solution to someone's life.

Reiki During Pregnancy

Reiki is beneficial to all age groups, even for those who are not born yet. Pregnant women who practice Reiki can extend their love to their unborn child by laying their hands upon their belly. By doing so, they help mothers to allow the Reiki energies that are abound within them, to be transferred to their baby.

Some Reiki practitioners even believe that if a pregnant woman practices Reiki, the baby will also be in vibrational alignment with the energies of Reiki too. This means that a child could be born with the gifts that Reiki offers, setting it up for a very pleasant and healthy life - a beautiful gift for any mother to give her child!

Reiki for Children

Reiki is a non-invasive healing system. This makes it a great choice for children, allowing you to help them deal with the growing pains they encounter (physical and emotional) in a way that is both easy on the child and you.

It has been found that children are extremely receptive to Reiki's positive effects too, and they normally welcome the processes of Reiki with little to no opposition.

The treatments for children are given in the same manner as they are for adults. The Reiki hand placements are identical, but the sessions are briefer. This is because Reiki energy flows through children a lot quicker than it does in adults. Children do not suffer from the emotional blockages that adults have, which leads to a quicker, more effective Reiki session.

Attuning Children

Although babies can very easily be attuned to Reiki, they cannot practice it. This is because the application of Reiki requires more than just energy reception (something babies excel at). Reiki, in order to be used, requires maturity and intention. So, children under six years of age are normally unable to practice Reiki.

However, children older than this, ideally between the ages five to twelve, can not only be vibrationally aligned to Reiki, but can practice it effectively too. With practice, supervision, and commitment, a child in this age range can (often easier than an adult) be successfully attuned to Reiki Level I (there will be more on the Reiki levels later in the book).

It is also **very important** to note that children who practice Reiki should be trained to not lay their hands upon their uninitiated classmates. This is because children that do not practice Reiki will be unfamiliar, unappreciative, and most likely fearful of having another child lay hands upon them. This fear can cause blockages in energy in both the Reiki practicing child and the recipient.

Reiki practicing children should be encouraged to practice their Reiki on themselves, stuffed animals, siblings, and their pets. As discussed later in this chapter, practicing Reiki on pets is a harmless process because animals are more than attuned to what energy they are willing to accept or reject. Therefore, letting your child practice Reiki on your pet is a relatively harmless procedure.

Reiki for Seniors

Reiki is most certainly suitable for people of all ages. But since Reiki is specifically good at alleviating pain, the elderly seem to gravitate toward the healing art.

Alzheimer patients (a demographic that makes up a lot of seniors) are particularly receptive to Reiki. This in itself is amazing because due to their conditions, Alzheimer patients normally find it next to impossible to apply alternative therapies.

But, Reiki allows these types of patients to access the powers of the healing art in such an easy way that the mental blocks of the condition are next to none.

As children grow and mature, they naturally become less dependent on their parents/guardians.

This independence is both natural and healthy; a result of growth.

However, if a young adult or middle-aged individual encounters a disease or illness that robs them of their independence, influencing them to seek help because they cannot manage on their own, they meet this situation with reluctance.

They would outwardly fight the circumstances, with comments like "I can manage," or "I'm ok." The loss of independence is often a fear that leads to some people not seeking professional medical assistance until things have escalated to a stage past help.

Many elderly people, however, understand that they can no longer be independent. They realize and come to terms with the fact that their lives will be easier with help, than without.

Reiki and Pets

The number of people that seek alternative therapies for their animals, is rising. An increasing number of people are shying away from relying solely on veterinarians, and instead are opting for therapies such as Reiki, Shiatsu, etc.

Animal lovers are sensitive to their pets and their illnesses. These owners wish to find therapies that not only help bring health to their animals, but are preventative too.

Reiki can truly fill this need for an effective treatment that offers holistic outcomes.

Using the energy systems of Reiki, animals can be healed quickly, effectively, and the risk of any adverse effects is next to nothing. In most cases of animals and Reiki, when the animal has had enough, they will instigate a break in the session by simply walking away.

Here is how Reiki is beneficial to animals:
- Accelerates healing of physical injuries
- Brings more calmness to the animal
- An energy practice creates a bond between animal and owner, one that improves the relationship

Haters and Skeptics

As with any new undertaking in life, when we start, we are not only skeptical ourselves, but we often have to deal with the skepticism of others too.

And more often than not, it is the skepticism of others that can lead to us quit a new endeavor, more so than our own doubts.

My advice to you regarding this is to have tunnel vision. Choose a goal or target (like learning Reiki) and focus on that solely. Do not allow the dispersions of others to sway you from your objective. Learn the art, use the art, and then - only then - can you, or should you, even really start to analyze something.

Reiki Responds Uniquely to Each Individual
Reiki is not a system that discriminates. The system treats imbalance.

There are many benefits derived from Reiki, but the results of treatments can vary as the result of several different factors:

- How many treatments or sessions of Reiki did the recipient partake in?
- What stage of the illness was the person at before starting Reiki?
- Did the recipient come into the process with expectations that were unrealistic or too high?
- How receptive was the recipient in allowing Reiki to heal their body?

Belief and Receptivity

Reiki works whether or not a person believes in it. The system works because it operates on certain universal laws of energy—laws that, much like those of gravity, cannot be broken.

However, if a person is not open to Reiki — in any way, shape or form — the energies and effects of Reiki will have a hard time getting past the blocks inside the individual. This is the real reason why some people who truly believe that Reiki will work, eventually feel let down, especially when Reiki seems to have no effect on them.

On the flip side, a skeptic that might not even consciously believe in the system may try Reiki and reap massive benefits, simply because subconsciously they were ready to receive Reiki.

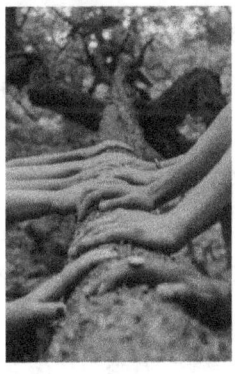

Reiki Benefits Everyone

Regardless of where you come from, Reiki is for you.

The art of Reiki is not one reserved only for the wealthy, educated, or spiritually evolved. Reiki is available to anyone who desires to open themselves to the system. The true 'cost of admission' is belief and embracing Reiki into yourself.

Treating Root Causes

Reiki needs to be used consistently. If used hastily, it will only bring short term effects of healing. But to enjoy long term effects, the healing system of Reiki must be applied continually.

Benefits of Reiki

Reiki will benefit you by empowering you in the following ways:

- Reiki reduces anxiety
- Stresses, something that is associated with long-term suffering, can be eradicated through the use of Reiki
- Reiki is safe to practice as opposed to some conventional health practices
- Reiki allows foods to be purified before consuming them by cleaning the energy associated with the food we are consuming
- Reiki energy is effective in helping people deal with grief
- Reiki both heals and can help free us of our emotional wounds
- Reiki allows us to let go of the negatives in life - people, wounds, and experiences

- Reiki helps us to effectively manifest. This makes the system great for goal setting and goal achieving

Chapter 6: The Third Eye; Background And History

The term the "Third Eye" is a relatively modern one – which explains a lot of those New Age associations that the term may bring to mind. However, the idea behind the concept is a very old one indeed and references can be found relating to the idea right back to our ancestor's earliest days – across most imaginable or recorded civilizations. In most traditions, the Third Eye was considered a symbol of enlightenment and closely linked with belief that it is possible to transcend physical sensations and the boundaries that they impose on our perception of the world.

References can be found to the concept of the Third Eye across many cultures. In ancient China it was better known as the "Mind's Eye" and there were many practices devoted to the development and training of this organ. These training techniques involved the individual meditating with their eyes closed and focusing clearly on the Third, or minds, eye while adopting specific poses that were believed to help improve the "vibration" of the Third Eye, opening it with the aim of connecting with the same vibrations emanating from the universal energy field.

Images, Art and the Third Eye

Symbolism has been used throughout history to denote the Third Eye as a concept. In some representations the eye takes the form of exactly that, an eye placed in the center of the forehead. However, in many traditions a pine-cone has come to symbolize the Third Eye. This symbol can be found in many cultures, including that of Ancient Egypt. At first glance, with whichever eye you choose to use, this may seem an odd symbol and there is certainly something oddly coincidental about the choice of the pine-cone. The Pineal Gland, whether or not this was known to ancient cultures, is

roughly the shape of a pine-cone (hence the name given to it by modern science.
Whilst it's possible that in some cultures ancient pathologists or priests were aware of the shape of this gland it seems unlikely that all of the depictions are the result of dissections. Depictions of the Third Eye (or its equivalent) which illustrate it as a pine-cone can be found in cultures as diverse as Ancient Egypt, ancient Assyria, ancient Mexican cultures and the European Greek and Roman civilizations.
In all of these cultures the symbol appears to relate to both enlightenment and immortality. This latter seems to be a similar concept to that which Descartes later gave the Pineal Gland when describing it as the "seat of the soul". As a symbol, pine-cones are also interesting in that not only do the trees that bear them appear to be immortal, or evergreen, but also they are some of the most ancient surviving species of plant on the planet,

predating flowering plants by many millennium.

The Links between the Pineal Gland and Third Eye

The Pineal Gland may also be referred to as the "pineal body" or the epiphysis cerebri. It is a simple, pea-sized structure but this small structure has some amazing qualities. The Pineal Gland produces several "chemicals" in the body and it is considered important by psychologists as these "natural happy drugs" can have a profound effect on both mood and on personality. Modern day theosophists, and those who study the esoteric, are also keen fans of the gland. For these groups it seems to provide a physical manifestation within the brain of the ancient concept of the Third Eye. For this group it is considered to be the most powerful source of energy and enlightenment that we possess and also responsible for psychic abilities of every kind. This group also argue that a closed Third Eye is responsible for negative emotions, including cynicism, anger, envy and lack of belief (in both the spiritual and the self). This argument has plenty of basis in fact, given that without a fully functioning Pineal Gland, the chemicals our bodies need to regulate mood, in a positive way, are absent.

The Third Eye is viewed as a gateway to developing and improving our psychic abilities and helps to improve the performance of our Sixth Chakra. Opening the Third Eye and bringing the Sixth Chakra to its fullest potential are often equated with the skills of the psychic and the clairvoyant. Active, and well developed, the Pineal Gland appears to promote both creativity, imagination and also to help to remember our dreams more clearly. It has also been linked to the ability to control our dreams (known as lucid dreaming) and to awake, or develop, precognition in many different forms. The Pineal Gland does, in fact, seem to become active during the night, particularly at the times when we normally dream. Usually, our dreams are at their most active between 01:00 am and 16:00 am and the Pineal Gland has been observed to become most active in average individuals at this time.

Science and Hallucinogenic Drugs

When it comes to natural "happy drugs" there's a lot of dispute about the role that the Pineal Gland plays. While it is well established that the gland is responsible for the production of melatonin, recent research suggests that it may well be secretly supplying a more hard-core drug to our system. The drug in question is "dimethyltryptamine", and it appears that the Pineal Gland may be able to secrete this hallucinogenic naturally in the body.

In recent years the drug has been found to be present in a wide range of both plant and animal species. Its natural production in humans is now established, but the purpose, the amounts and the "why" is as yet unclear.

Some researchers believe that the drug can (and does) flood the body during the process of birth and also that of death. Additionally there have been suggestions that this natural drug is present in the body during the 13th week of pregnancy, although clear evidence of this is yet to be fully established. If this latter fact is true, another strange coincidence with ancient teachings may be found in relation to the Pineal Gland – the 13th week of pregnancy is traditionally considered in Tibetan Buddhism to be the point at which the soul enters the physical body!

Scientifically, the Pineal Gland is, in fact, a real "Third" eye; the tissues from which it is formed are the same as those from which the retina is composed. As in animals which have a more clearly defined Third Eye the Pineal Gland remains sensitive to light in humans and although the mechanism of how this works is not fully understood, scientists have established that light levels have a direct impact on this small, deeply hidden gland!

The Faulty Third Eye Dilemma

We all have a Pineal Gland and the chances are that yours is working! Certainly it would be impossible to sleep at all (ever) if the Pineal Gland we possess was not functioning. Although some people suffer from insomnia from time to time, the condition is nearly always related to other health problems or results from issues not related to the Pineal Gland. In most individuals the Pineal Gland is fine!

However, some people seem to possess psychic and clairvoyant qualities naturally, or have learned to "open" their Third Eye effectively. While everybody has a Pineal Gland, not everybody appears to have psychic abilities.

As mentioned earlier in this book, the Pineal Gland is one of those parts of the body that is sensitive to calcium deposits. This process, calcification, can happen in soft tissue in different parts of the body but is most commonly seen in arteries, heart valves and the Pineal Gland itself. The condition is caused by imbalances in vital vitamins (vitamin K2 deficiency and vitamin D overdose) and these imbalances can alter the way in which our body absorbs calcium (essential for bone development) and allow deposits to accumulate in the wrong areas.

Unfortunately modern lifestyles and our modern diet are not, despite what we may believe, what we were built for. Our bodies, including that small pea-sized gland, have evolved over tens of thousands of years and have not adapted for either the way in which we now live or the food that we commonly eat. This, in turn, means that both our lifestyle and diet can lead to poor nutrition and general health, and these factors greatly increase the risk of calcification. Although this calcification is actually a natural part of the aging process, calcification of the Pineal

Gland seems to happen disproportionately early and is common by our teenage years, developing to a much greater extent by the time we are only in our forties. In some cases the gland simply begins to shrivel and wither away, retaining limited function in either its physical or psychic senses. This goes a long way towards explaining why so many people believe that they are not (or could not be) psychic in anyway. There is, however, some good news; opening your Third Eye and de-calcifying your Pineal Gland are perfectly possible! In the rest of this book we'll explore the best techniques to achieving exactly that!

Chapter 7: The Benefits Of Reiki Healing

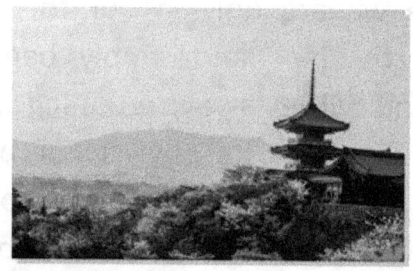

Because Reiki is a healing technique, therapists use it to channel energy to their patients through touch. They are activating the natural healing process that is already inside patients' body in order to help re-balance their emotional and physical well-being.

Treatment like this makes the patients feel as if there is a glowing radiance flowing through them and around them. It is a simple and natural method of healing that is going to complement other techniques that may be used by the patient's doctor or any other therapeutic techniques that they may be applying to their life.

Reiki sessions will take place with the patient fully clothed as the practitioner places his or her hands on various parts of the patient's body.

It's important to understand that Reiki practice balances a patient on every level. Patients may find that they feel refreshed and at peace after they experience a Reiki session. Below I'm listing some of the crucial healing benefits of Reiki:

Reiki promotes of health and well-being through energy healing

It can help with pain management because patients are using their energy to help reduce the pain.

Patients experience mental clarity because they are being forced to push all the negativity aside to focus on the positive energy.

While pushing out all the negativity, patients will experience a release in tension and stress.

Patients using Reiki will see that their depression is relieved.

Patients using Reiki will also notice that they have a lower anxiety level.

It helps patients to experience a state of relaxation through energy healing.

Due to the relaxation that the patients will experience, they will also notice that they are able to sleep better.

With energetic healing, patients will notice that their digestive system runs smoother than it did before.

Without all of the negativity running around inside the patients' head, they are able to have higher self-esteem.

Reiki helps to heighten patients' self-awareness because they will understand what is going on in their body.

With Reiki, patients can find support for substance abuse and get help recovering from it.

It helps promote harmony and balance because it is enhancing the body's natural healing ability.

Reiki helps get rid of energy blocks and helps promote the natural balance found between the mind, body, and spirit.

Reiki helps clean the body of toxins while supporting the immune system. Because many patients find that they are in a fight-or-flight phase so much, their bodies tend to return to their natural balance. With Reiki, our bodies are reminded to shift into self-healing mode.

Patients' self-healing ability will be able to start so that they can return to the natural state. Even if patients do not get to this natural state instantly, they will be pushed in the proper direction. This helps blood pressure and heart rate to improve.

Reiki helps with spiritual growth and emotional cleansing because it addresses the entire person instead of just addressing specific symptoms.

Chapter 8: History Of Reiki

REIKI is an old Tibetan type of healing. (pronounced Ray Key, it's a Japanese term and that means Universal life force energy).REIKI was found in the center of the nineteenth century by Dr. Mikao Usui.

Dr. Usui was the top of a Christian Faculty in Kyoto, in Japan. His pupils told him 1 day that they'd not heard of the recovery methods utilized by Jesus Christ., they requested Dr. Usui in case he can do this particular healing type for them. Regrettably Dr. Usui didn't have the information for the students of his, and with that he resigned as head of the Faculty, and also set out on a journey to discover the answers.

He traveled to America to learn and also received a greater degree in Theology in the Faculty of Chicago. Next, he traveled to Japan to train in the healings of the Chinese Buddha and Sutra, and then on to Tibet in which he learned Sanskrit (the early language of The Tibetan and India) Lotus Sutra. It was right here that he discovered the answers he was searching for, the solutions to healing methods of Christ. He required the empowerment now.

He went to Japan and climbed the Holy Mountain of Kuri Yama, wherever he fasted as well as meditated for twenty one days, to identify the reality of the Sanskrit technique. He placed twenty one stones before him and every day which passed by he will eliminate one stone. Throughout the time of his on the mountain Dr.Usui examine the sutras, meditated and also sang. Dr.Usui did this for the twenty one days though almost nothing occurred until the really last day. As the morning started, though it was nonetheless silent dim and saw a brilliant light move towards him with a little pace. As it came closer to him it grew larger on hit and size him during the temple.

He watched a lot of small bubbles in pink, lilac and most of the shades of the rainbow. Dr. Usui believed he'd died when a fantastic white light came out before him, he looked up and also discovered the popular Sanskrit symbols before him glowing in Gold, he said' Yes I remember'. This was the development of the Usui process of REIKI.

When he returned to truth, the sunshine was uploaded with the skies, he was loaded with passion, he felt full of daily life, energy and strength, and though he'd fasted on the Holy Mountain for twenty one days he ran on the hill. This was the very first magic.

From the rush of his down the mountain, he stubbed the toe of his. He held it with the hands of his and in a couple of mins the bleeding as well as the pain stopped. This was the next miracle.

In the haste of his to get on the mountain Dr. Usui knocked the toe of his. He wrapped the hands of his close to the foot of his for a couple of moments the bleeding as well as the pain both disappeared. This was the next miracle.

Since he'd not eaten in twenty one days he was starved, he came across an Inn on the roadside and purchased a big Japanese breakfast, the innkeeper advised him not to consume such a big food after fasting for so very long. But Dr. Usui managed to complete the meal without any problem. This was the final miracle.

The inn keeper's granddaughter was definitely struggling a number of times with a toothache. Dr. Usui placed the hands of his gently on the inflamed face of her and she started to feel happier right away. She ran to grandfather and also clarified he was no typical monk. This particular healing was the 4th miracle of the morning.

Dr Usui returned to the abbey of his in Kyoto to cure the folks from the Beggar City and also the slums. During his 7 years treating individuals in the shelter he noticed the same faces were going back to him. He questioned them, exactly why had they not moved on and begin a brand new lifestyle. The individuals revealed to him it had been better to begin begging as work was way too hard. Dr. Usui was surprised by this, and discovered he'd forgotten a thing of great value throughout the healings which was teaching the beggars gratitude

Dr. Chikiro Hayashi, one of Dr. Usui's closest colleagues evolved into the next REIKI Grand Master in the series of the tradition. He ran the own private Clinic of his in Tokyo until 1940. He will treat unusual and severe cases. In serious cases REIKI will be administered around the clock

Throughout 1900 a lady named Hawayo Takata came into this world on the island of Hawaii, the parents of her were Japanese, and was a citizen of the United States. She was widowed with 2 children that are young. Throughout 1935 the path of her led her to REIKI. She was being affected by a serious illness in the moment, when an internal voice told her to seek healing in Japan.

Ms. Takata went to Japan, to find healing. She was resting on the operating table every time a voice spoke to her, explaining that there was clearly no requirement to proceed through with the operation. She requested the physician regarding various other strategies for therapy and also he advised her going to Dr. Hayashi's REIKI Clinic. After, there, REIKI was put on to Ms. Takata every day by 2 providers and within a few months, she was to total health.

Hawayo Takata evolved into a pupil of Dr. Hayashi's for annually after which returned to Hawaii with her 2 daughters. She was launched a Master by Dr. Hayashi as he visited Hawaii in 1938 and she succeeded him as Grand Master in 1941. She lived, healed as well as qualified REIKI Masters. On the 11th of December in1980, Hawayo Takata passed away, making twenty two REIKI Masters throughout the USA as well as Canada.

Chapter 9: The Definition Of Reiki:

Reiki is a Japanese word, made up by two syllables, kanji (Japanese syllables):
REI – universal, love, divine, cosmic, vital;
KI – energy, movement, vibration.
By combining these two syllables we can understand the true meaning of Reiki: Universal Energy, Spiritual Energy, Vital Universal Force, Energy of Unconditional Love etc. Even if the word Reiki is Japanese, the Reiki energy is Universal.

Modern science came to the conclusion that the Universe is made up of vibrations and waves. Reiki is one of them, the vibration of Love and Harmony.

REIKI is a Japanese natural energetic technique in which the hands are used for guiding the energy as a connector to the Vital Energy of the Universe. The purpose of this energy is to return our vitality, to relax us, to reduce stress and to improve the quality of our lives through the development of our personalities and our energetical, physical, emotional, mental and spiritual balance.

All living creatures have the innate ability to restore their health in a natural way. The human body has all the necessary resources to function, to protect itself and to regenerate through its physiological processes, its immune and hormone system, etc. Our ancestors observed the laws of the Universe and lived in harmony with them. They knew and used the intelligence of the body and those of the laws of nature and these pieces of information were imprinted and transmitted to future generations. Sometimes humans act instinctively based on this innate and ancestral intelligence.

For instance, we place our hands instinctively on the spot that hurts, as a reflex inherited from our ancestors. Reiki is a natural method that teaches us to use our hands to attract vitality and balance in our bodies by accessing the Universal energy and (unconditional) Love. Humans and all living creatures receive Reiki through its three forms:

Reiki, as the energy that drives life (natural vitality),

Reiki, as a spiritual activity (the power of the soul),

Reiki, as a self-healing method (the power of the physical body).

Reiki works because it is energy received from the Heavens; it is called Universal energy and it is radiant. Although it is an invisible energy, those who practice Reiki can sometimes see it.

Reiki Energy helps all living things to live in balance. Because it is a natural energy, it helps life and evolution. Compare this to "artificial" energies (Roentgen, cobalt, isotopes) which, if used in excess, may harm living organisms. The human being is the supreme creation, benefitting from individual consciousness and therefore has access to more energies/information than other living creatures and can use these energies for its wellbeing. It is only because of illusions, materialism, upsets and fears that we have a tendency to forget the gifts received from the Universe.

If we would like to know how to become channels for the Reiki energy we have to eliminate our limited thinking and be open to Nature and the Universe, who accept us naturally, without reserve and offer us the power of Reiki. This is important in order to be healthy and balanced in all aspects of life. When practicing Reiki we may feel some uncertainty at first, but we will observe the results as we progress and we will come to offer Reiki to the sick without hesitation or fear.

Student observation: "I do not believe in energies and auras. How can I influence energies?"

15-18 years ago my answer to this question was very simplistic, as the information to which I had access at that time was limited. I used to hang on to words and explain this using a string of ideas which seemed logical to me in terms of the physics taught in school: matter is formed by atoms which have a nucleus (protons and neutrons with positive charge) around which electrons are moving. So because we are talking about movement/gravitation/vibration; I concluded that because there is movement, there is energy.

In biology we were taught that at a cellular Level, mitochondria transform the ingested food into energy.

I also knew from physics that nothing ever gets lost, everything is transformed. So, if there is vibration and transformation there are also ways through which these can be influenced and harmonized.

Today we have access to a large amount of information and research about the meaning of energy, energetic fields, consciousness and Divinity. This book, however, has another purpose as I didn't set out to write a scientific book on this subject. But for those who are curios, skeptical or those who like me are not willing to settle for pure statements and need more information, I am going to briefly present the connection with these scientific approaches. You may then independently continue to research if you wish to do so.

The book contains references on how to achieve a state of balance at all Levels and less scientific arguments, as Reiki balances the communication between the two cerebral hemispheres and develops emotional intelligence. Read the book both with your mind and your heart in order to fully understand its message.

Quantum mechanics and quantum physics offer an interesting approach and describe the behavior of matter at the atomic and subatomic Level and explain processes for which neither Newtonian physics nor the theory of electromagnetism offer sufficient or complete information.

Classic Newtonian physics is based on the observation of objects, on day-to-day experiments that can be repeatedly verified, tested and proven, therefore reaching the understanding of physical behavior. Biologically speaking the physical body is analyzed as an ensemble of organs, each organ having separate and well-determined functions; the body should thus work as a "precise and exact Swiss watch", everything unfolding according to a perfect pre-established mechanism. In reality things are different, both in nature and in the human body. The information/energy that cells are bearing is being ignored. The importance and intelligence of cells, which are the basis of the body and the organs, are not being recognized.

When physicists started analyzing the subatomic Level of matter the Newtonian laws and theories proved limited. The concepts of quantum mechanics started being developed between 1926 and 1935. Here are prominent names of those who further developed these concepts up to the integration of the notion of consciousness into quantum physics: Max Born, Erwin Schrödinger, Werner von Heisenberg (uncertainty principle, establishes the limits between the theories of classical physics and those of quantum mechanics), Pascual Jordan, Wolfgang Pauli, Niels Bohr (the Bohr-Bohm theory), Paul Dirac, John von Neumann, Stephen Hawking, Nassim Haramein, Amit Goswami.

Quantum mechanics is based on mathematical formalism which describes physical phenomena through vectors and space operators and its measurements are not based on determinism. For instance, particles do not move on well-determined orbits, but are characterized by probability. In time a series of interpretations were developed, regarding the measurement process of a subatomic particle, as there are always additional uncertainties generated by probability. Niels Bohr said: "We can only know the probable position of a moving particle, therefore by extension, we can only know its probable destination; we can never know with absolute certainty where it will go."

The first great scission in quantum physics came about through the dispute between Albert Einstein and Niels Bohr. In the theory of relativity through the relativity formula $E = mc2$, Albert Einstein surprised the scientific community of his time, proving that time and space are not separate entities and that they are not only connected to each other but are part of a whole called the time-space continuum. Most of his contributions to physics are linked to the theory of special relativity that combines mechanics with electromagnetism and to the theory of general relativity that extends the principle of the relativity of disorderly motion. Lots of books on quantum physics mention that Albert Einstein supported the idea according to which "the field is the sole governing agency of the particle." This is a fact confirmed by outlooks, cultures and oriental philosophies for thousands of years: „spirit shapes matter". Among Einstein's contributions we count his quantum theory of the monoatomic ideal gas and although the quantum theory was one of the immediate consequences of his scientific contributions Einstein never agreed with the interpretations brought to this theory by Niels Bohr and Werner Heisenberg.

Einstein had heated discussions with the great physicist Niels Bohr about the uncertainty principle that would arise from the probabilistic character of mathematical descriptions contained in quantum physics. He wrote the following in a letter addressed to physicist Max Born in 1962, referring to Bohr's uncertainty principle: "I am convinced that God does not play dice". To which Bohr replied: "Then stop telling God what to do with them." According to the theory of relativity (deterministic theory) dices seem unpredictable, however knowing the details of their motion one should be able to determine how they will fall.

Einstein died without acknowledging Bohr's quantum theory but contributed to it through his work.

Niels Bohr, a Danish physicist, created the first model of the quantic nature of the atom (bearing his name) and brought interesting contributions to understanding the subatomic structure and quantum mechanics.

The physicist and neuropsychologist David Bohm introduced the holistic approach according to which the world cannot be analyzed as separate subunits and so, the fragmented approach was replaced with a unifying one that integrates the observer (consciousness) into the physical reality of the world. In the Universe everything is part of an immense continuum. Bohm declared that in the Universe each thing is part of the Whole, retaining however its unique characteristics. Bohm also stated that the Universe is only energy and potential.

The History of REIKI

A lot has been written about the history of Reiki. There are two mainstream versions and their supporters express their opinion often too vehemently. Traditionally information is passed on verbally from Master to disciple and not a lot of written information is offered. Since the history of Reiki is mainly based on the oral transmission of information, several versions have emerged.

I would rather approach an integrative view of history, explaining the documented history of Mikao Usui Sensei and Reiki, telling the Reiki "legend" from which I am going to extract a few examples from the version presented by Ms Takata, with modifications that were attributed to her.

Even if healing practices involving the hands existed in most of the ancient cultures Reiki was elaborated by Mikao Usui Sensei, who was born in Japan in 1865, in the village of Taniai (today the city of Mijama). His father, Uzaemon Cunetane, was a military commander; his mother came from the Kavaai family. Usui studied different oriental practices without ever becoming a monk.

Going through various life experiences Usui searched for and found the meaning of life, „Anshin Ritsumei", meaning "Your spirit being fully at peace, being aware of what you should do with your life, totally undisturbed." In order to achieve this, he meditated for 21 days in February and March 1922 on the mountain of Kurama, about 12 km away from Kyoto, where he discovered the connection and resonance with the Reiki vibration. In some books/histories it is mentioned that Usui originally began teaching the TEATE method, meaning "healing with the hands". The name came from what he was doing, and not from past teachings. This method preceded the USUI REIKI RYOHO method (meaning "The Reiki Usui healing method").

In April 1922 Mikao Usui founded the USUI REIKI RYOHO Gakkai organization. At first, in order to practice Reiki, disciples lived close to their Master and Reiki was transmitted from the aura of the Master to the aura of the disciples. Initiations were not performed as we know them today. The Reiki symbols were introduced later by Mikao Usui, with the purpose of making Reiki practice easier. Even today not all symbols are used in Gakkai.

I like telling the following stories from the "legend" passed on by Ms Takata. They may not be real, but because I was taught these stories and I grew with them, I like telling them. I assume responsibility and take the risk of introducing these elements into the history of Reiki that I teach at my courses:

a) When Mikao Usui decided to climb Mount Kurama he only took with him 21 pebbles, one for each day. Every day, at sunrise, he used to throw a pebble. On the last day, when he only had one pebble left, while meditating, Mikao Usui was surrounded by light and he reached a state of happiness. When he recovered from this state he was aware that he had received that for which he had been searching for such a long time and that he had entered the vibration of Reiki energy. Coming down the mountain, Mikao Usui hurt one of his legs and instinctively put his hand on the wounded spot; he noticed that his hand got very warm, that the bleeding stopped and the healing process began. This for him was the first sign that the thing he had received from the Universe really worked.

At the foot of the mountain there was a pilgrims' shelter where he stopped to eat. The woman who brought him food had a strong toothache. Usui asked for permission to place his hands near her face, close to her teeth. She agreed and after a few minutes of holding his palms close to her face the pain decreased.

b) Following these "happenings" Mikao Usui settled down in Tokyo and opened a retreat where he treated people using Reiki. Mikao Usui decided to introduce the five Reiki principles to all those who practice Reiki.

Now back to the real history. In September 1923 after the earthquake in Japan, Usui and his disciples were assisting victims. This is how Usui and Reiki became known. Officers of the Japanese navy found out about Reiki and Usui and invited him to teach them Reiki. Some of the navy officers were taught up to the Shinpiden Level. Usui passed away on the 9th of March 1926, but his method was passed on by approximately 2000 people practicing Reiki and by the 21 Reiki Shinpiden. The names of 12 of the 21 Shinpinden disciples are known to us.

In 1927 Gakkai builds Mikao Usui's funeral monument in Tokyo, inside the Saiho-ji

Temple. Gakkai is the only organization that is allowed to build monuments or commemorative plaques for Usui. Gakkai is still active to this day. It is an organization with limited access and has only 500 members.

Usui Reiki Ryoho, currently called Dento Reiki, is practiced only in Japan, and the Reiki lines outside of Japan are called Western/Occidental Reiki.

Chujiro Hayashi, a former Navy officer and military doctor, and a graduate of the Naval Japanese Academy came in contact with Reiki through Admiral Taketomi, who was Usui's disciple. In 1925 Hayashi met Mikao Usui. Some versions of the history of Reiki mention that Usui asked Hayashi to do some research on Reiki and to develop the techniques of Reiki and the Reiki practice. After Usui's death, Hayashi left Gakkai and formed the Hayashi Reiki Kenkyukai Institute, where he continued his research.

Ms. Takata was talking about the clinic opened by C. Hayashi where Reiki practitioners were working as a group, as volunteers for a year, treating patients staying in the clinic. This was compulsory work experience required to reach a more advanced Level in Reiki (Okuden). Hawayo Takata came to this clinic as a patient in 1935.

Chujiro Hayashi left this world on the 11th of May 1940.

Hawayo Takata, was of Japanese origin and was born on the 24th of December 1900 on the island of Kauai in Hawaii. She became a widow at a young age. Because of her health issues she left Hawaii and went to Tokyo to have surgery. She discussed with her doctor if there are any other options apart from surgery. He then recommended Hayashi's clinic where Ms. Takata got well within a few months. Seeing the benefits of this technique Ms. Takata wanted to learn Reiki, so in 1973 she received Level II and went back to Hawaii where she opened a Reiki clinic.

Chujiro Hayashi visited her in 1938 in Hawaii. He stayed for six months and seeing the results she had achieved he granted her the Level of Reiki teacher on the 21st of February 1938.

Ms. Takata is considered to be the founder of Occidental Reiki and thanks to her it became known in the USA. This happened during adverse historic conditions when Japan and the USA were in conflict and anyone/anything of Japanese origins was being regarded as suspicious. After the December 1941 attack on Pearl Harbor the anti-Japanese sentiment in Americans ran high. It is, therefore, understandable that Ms. Takata "adapted" Reiki to be better suited to the Occidental way, introducing elements of Christianity in Reiki and giving up certain practical exercises.

She used to start Reiki courses with the introduction of the energy of the Universe which she defined as infinite energy, a force descending from the Source/Creator that is surrounding us. She named this method USUI SHIKI RYOHO (meaning the "Usui-style healing method "). Due to the conditions of that time Ms Takata simplified some of the Reiki exercises taught by Usui and Hayashi and in order to be able to practice certain Reiki exercises she obtained a diploma in massage. After the bombardment of Japan by the USA in 1945 Ms. Takata no longer had ties with Japan. Hawayo Takata held Reiki courses for over 40 years in the USA and Canada and during her final years she trained 22 Masters.

The title of Master was granted in Japan only to those who achieved Illumination. However, Takata started using this title in 1970 when she started offering initiations for the Level of Reiki teacher/ teacher. Therefore we need to clarify that a Reiki Master in the West is not necessarily someone who has attained illumination.

Ms. Takata left this world at 80 years of age, on the 25th of December 1980. I feel the deepest respect for Ms Takata who had the courage to promote and practice Reiki during a very difficult period in history.

There are different versions in the USA and in Japan regarding the course of Reiki after Ms. Takata's death. However, Reiki, if it truly is Reiki, works the same, both in the West, East and in Japan.

Chapter 10: Principles Of Reiki

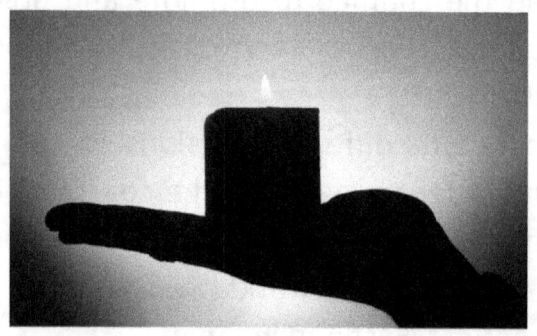

Reiki operates on Five Principles that Dr. Usui discovered in his meditation practices. These five principles are a way to release the stories and energies that your mind tells you that create suffering in your daily life.

Generally, daily activities aren't meant to cause stress and anxiety. It is the mind and the beliefs that stay in the mind which create that stress and anxiety. My unraveling those limitations, your mind can let go and you can have a sense of balance and peace in your life and in your thoughts.

These five principles allow you to improve your actions and thought patterns day to day and moment by moment. Your conscious thoughts and actions over time become your natural way of thinking and being. That is the importance of the five Reiki principles.

The five Reiki principles are:

For all of today, I will not worry

For all of today, I will not be angry

For all of today, I will work honestly

For all of today, I will be grateful for my blessings

For all of today, I will be kind to all living things

These principles can become important in your everyday life. To incorporate the principles, into your life, you can say them aloud like mantras. You can use them in your daily meditations, or write them out and post them on a wall, or at your desk at work.

Each individual feels a different resonance with the five principles and will gain a different meaning from them. These meanings and resonances can change over time. When you first start working with these principles, they might carry a certain resonance, and then over time they might begin to mean something new to you.

If the traditional principles in Reiki don't resonate with you, trying different wording. Some other popular variations include:

Just for today, I will trust

Just for today, I will love

Just for today, I will be true to myself and others

Just for today, I will give thanks for my blessings

Just for today I will be kind to every living thing

Another practice for getting in touch with these principles and making them a part of your life is to hold their intention and really feel what it feels like. You can meditate and focus on the principles while lying down or sitting up.

Try closing your eyes and repeating each of the principles out loud, several times. You can also practice saying them in your mind and use whatever method feels the most comfortable. Take the time to sit with each principle and really feel its intention and its meaning wash over you and through you.

As you perform these exercises with the five Reiki principles, you might want to document the different experiences, feelings, and sensations that come up for you. Keeping a journal can help you see your personal growth and progression with the Reiki principles as you keep including them into your healing and your life.

For all of today, I will not worry

Worry as an emotion can be helpful. Worry can help work through some situations in a healthy way. When worry occurs in excess or occurs frequently, it can become problematic. Anytime an emotion becomes problematic it impacts the body, mind, and spirit.

When you worry, your mind is focused on the future. Although a small amount of worry can be helpful in taking action in the present, excessive worry can lead to anxiety, confusion, and stagnation. Being present in the moment is how you can be most effective. Through this principle, you will learn to trust in the wisdom of Reiki to guide you through life's ups and downs.

When you experience difficulty, those moments often leave to the most crucial points of development. Developing a fearful and worrisome mindset you will begin to see positive and neutral events only from a negative perspective. Releasing those beliefs will instead help you perceive situations from a more positive angle.

Be open to where life is leading you and enjoy the ride that is life. Life gives you ups and downs, be present for it all to empower yourself for growth and change. To really support this Reiki principle, make time in your day for activities that you enjoy. Surround yourself with people who resonate with a peaceful, happy energy. That energy will become a part of you as well.

For all of today, I will not be angry

The emotion of anger stems from a place where you feel like you have no control or a lack of power. When a perceived negative event occurs that you have a strong association with, the emotion may not be processed properly or released. The body stores the emotion rather than releasing it. When another even occurs that reminds you of the original event that anger resurfaces from where it was stored, only this time you have anger that is responding to both evens and is stronger, causing heightened reactions.

Over time, the emotions get stored up more and more, creating pressure. Then a simple trigger can result in an explosive reaction.

Part of working with Reiki energy and in healing yourself is in processing and releasing stored emotions in a constructive, healthy way. Anger is difficult to process in a healthy way because society teaches people from a young age that anger is negative and shouldn't be expressed.

If you experience anger, take a step back from the situation, then breathe into the anger. Become a witness to the even. From the viewpoint of being a witness you will be able to let that anger emotion pass through you rather than storing it for a later event.

Meditating on a daily basis on what the absence of anger feels like can help you process this emotion more effectively. Additionally, if you meditate on choosing to feel emotions that are a higher vibration than anger, you can help yourself default to more positive thought patterns rather than storing the anger.

When angry, taking deep breath after deep breath, and focusing on those breaths, can actually help you feel the release of the pressure that is built up from anger. Every person and every experience have a lesson for you. Approaching situations and people from a place of wanting to learn and being open to knowledge, you'll find that these lessons come easier. Responding to an event or a person in anger results in an incomplete lesson and you are more likely to relive that event with more intense energies and emotions.

For all of today, I will work honestly

In your heart of hearts, you know when you are being honest with yourself. When you aren't being honest, dissatisfaction becomes your body's way of showing you that you aren't being honest.

By not honoring your own dreams, passions, and talents, you lead a dishonest life. If you make decisions based on fear then you are definitely not being true to your soul or your heart.

The role you have to play is very important in this world. The role that each individual has to play in this world is important. The way you live and your actions make a difference in the lives of everyone that crosses your path. Assuming you don't have that impact does not serve yourself or the world. The impact you are here to make is guided by your dreams and desires. This helps you discover what the universe wants for you to accomplish. Honor yourself by following your dreams and live honestly.

For all of today, I will be grateful for my blessings

It is not uncommon to view events as good or bad. This is a result of the ego getting in the way. The soul or spirit, however, sees each event as an opportunity to grow and strengthen. Each experience brings you to a place that you can increase your awareness, and mindfulness.

Many people continue to search for external sources of pleasure, happiness, and gratification. It is the hope that these external sources will make you feel good and the mentality of 'I will be happy when...' becomes a thought at the forefront of the mind. It can be a hard lesson to learn that the true source of happiness comes from within.

You can start learning this and experiencing this by being grateful for your blessings every day. Be grateful now, in this moment, at this time and it will bring more positivity into your life. As you project this gratefulness and experience it, your environment will shift to match those changes.

Gratitude is a powerful intention. Gratitude raises the vibration of your body, mind, and spirit as well as bringing you insight and wisdom. Everyone, including you, has countless things to be grateful for. Defaulting to this Reiki principle is going to help you focus on your blessings and allow you to bring much more into your life.

Holding the intention of gratitude every day will have a dramatic effect on your life. You can even use Reiki to hold that intention of gratitude as well as one of the Three Pillars of Reiki, the Gassho, which will be discussed further along in this chapter.

When using Reiki to hold your intention of gratitude, you can place one hand on your third eye chakra at your brow and the other on the third eye chakra at the base of your skull.

For all of today, I will be kind to all living things

As previously touched on, the energetic frequency that you project or emanate will attract other things, people, jobs, and situations, that also resonate with that energy. Holding a high vibration will bring you to people and situations with similar high vibrations.

There is a study by Dr. Masuro Emoto where he researches the results of intentions with water. Negative intentions, like spoken words and thoughts, changed the molecular composition of the water in a less than appealing way. This was photographed at a molecular level to display the differences in how water exposed to negative intentions differed from water exposed to positive intentions. The human body is made up of eighty percent water. Focusing on intentions such as kindness and positivity stand to change your water composition on a molecular level and increase your energetic vibration. It keeps the body, mind, and spirit, healthy. The individuals that you encounter every day serve as mirrors into yourself. By keeping your energetic vibration high, the people you interact with start to reflect that as well.

It is your choice to life a life of peace, balance, and satisfaction. You have the power to create that life for yourself. Why pass that up?

Even Dr. Usui who discovered and performed Reiki, spent a great deal of his time in meditation and inner contemplation for personal and spiritual growth. He worked to increase his awareness to become a strong and effective conduit to channel Reiki energy through himself. Along with incorporating the five Reiki principles into your life and mentality, performing Reiki treatments on yourself every day will also make a difference. Release the limiting beliefs imposed on you by society and that you've put on yourself and your own world.

Along with the five Reiki principles, there are Three Pillars of Reiki that are going to improve your life, your vibration, and your environment. They will also help you connect more deeply with Reiki energy and healing.

The Three Pillars of Reiki are:
Gassho (Gash-Show)
Reiji-Ho (Ray-Gee-Hoe)
Chiryo (Chi-Rye-Oh)

These three Reiki pillars are going to help deepen your connection to Reiki energy. They are going to aid you in your work with the five Reiki Principles. More than that they are going to provide you with additional tools to help in your self-treatment sessions and with the work you do with clients.

The three Reiki Pillars are taught in the Reiki Level II course because they do include some more advanced techniques and sometimes employ the use of Reiki Symbols which are taught at Reiki Level II. However, you can adapt them and find ways to include them into your every day healing and Reiki practice without using the advanced Reiki symbols.

Gassho

Gassho is a type of Reiki meditation. The translation of Gassho is: two hands coming together. The Gassho meditation is meant to hold the intention of gratitude, focus, respect, connection, and balance to collective consciousness.

Dr. Usui's students were taught to place their hands in the Gassho position each morning and each night. Gassho helps to quiet and focus the mind during meditation. It can be incorporated into a meditation or be what you use to start your meditation to help you focus your mind.

The Gassho position is placing your hands palms together in the prayer position. Close your eyes and bring your awareness to the tips of your middle fingers. Any time your mind begins to wander, gently press your middle fingers together and allow the pressure to help you refocus your intention.

Traditionally, there are two different forms of Gassho. There is formal and informal. Formal Gassho is most commonly used in rituals such as religious services or formal gatherings. Formal Gassho is when you bring your hands together in the prayer position with your fingers pointing towards the sky. Your elbows should be raised with your forearms at an approximately 30-degree angle to the floor. Your fingertips should be level with your eyebrows but your hands should be around four inches from the tip of your nose. Focus your eyes on the tips of your middle fingers.

Mu-shin, which means No Mind, Gassho is a form of Gassho that is used for the purpose of greeting others. In this Gassho meditation, your hands are held together in the prayer position, however you'll want your fingers toughing with a little space between your palms. You'll want your elbows at a 45-degree angle to the floor and your hands four inches from the front of your face. Your fingertips should be just below your nose, lower than the formal Gassho. You can also perform Mu-shin Gassho with your hands positioned in front of the chest above the heart. Again, your eyes should be focused on the tips of your middle fingers.

The recommended amount of time for this meditation is to perform it for about fifteen to thirty minutes. If you find it beneficial, try doing this meditation each morning and each evening for a month. Take notes your experiences with Gassho and any changes you notice in your life.

The Gassho meditation should be performed while seated. Whenever a thought or emotion arises, watch them go by and pass through you, continuing on their way and refocus on your fingertips.

Some people find it beneficial to recite the five Reiki principles during a Gassho meditation. If your arms become uncomfortable, lower them down slightly, or put your hands in your lap. When you finish the meditation, send an intention of gratitude. If you need grounding, set your palms on the floor in front of you to end the session completely.

Reiji-Ho

The word Reiji in English means: indication of the Reiki energy. The word Ho means: technique. The Reiji-Ho pillar consists of three techniques that can be performed before each Reiki session. These can help with self-treatment sessions or sessions that are performed on others.

The three rituals of Reiji-Ho are going to align you more deeply with Reiki before you begin channeling it through your body. They are going to enhance each session that you give to yourself or perform on someone else by providing a more focused session.

Step One

The first step in Reiji-Ho is to hold your hands in the Gassho position in front of your chest, eyes closed.

Using the CKR and HSZSN Reiki symbols, ask for the Reiki energy to flow through you. If you do not know the Reiki symbols yet, in your mind, set the strong intention and desire calling on the Reiki energy to flow through you.

Repeat this request three times to shift your mind into that state.

If you are attuned to Reiki Level II, intone the CKR and SHK symbol to hold your intention. If you are not yet attuned to Reiki Level II, assert in your mind that you are holding that intention of Reiki energy flowing through you firmly in your mind.

Step Two

The first part to step two of Reiji-Ho is to ask for the balancing of your client/recipient, or yourself.

Next, you'll want to raise your hands to your third eye chakra at your brow while continuing to keep your hands in the Gassho position.

Set the intention that the Reiki energy will guide your hands to where Reiki energy is needed.

Step Three

Allow the Reiji-Ho technique to guide your hands. Allow your mind to detach from any desires or outcomes regarding the Reiki session you are about to perform. Open yourself up to receiving messages that will help guide you during the session. Let your hands move over your body or the body of your client. Let your intuition and Reiki guide you to where Reiki is needed. Once Reiji-Ho is complete, your hands will rest.

Place your hands back in the Gassho position again. Then proceed with the Reiki session as normal with hand positions.

It is up to your personal preference whether to discuss anything you find or see during a Reiki session with your clients or recipients.

Chiryo

The word Chiryo means: treatment. To perform Chiryo, you as the practitioner will place your dominant hand over your client's crown chakra. You can also perform Chiryo on yourself by placing your dominant hand over your own crown chakra during a self-treatment.

When you receive an intuitive indication that you should move your hands, begin to move your non-dominant hand over your body or your recipient's body. Allow your hand to follow the guidance you receive from the Reiki energy and your own intuition.

You'll want to keep placing your hands on the body as you are called, holding a position for as long as you are guided to. Chiryo can be performed as a treatment session on its own or as an added aspect to a Reiki session with the traditional hand positions.

Chapter 11: Body, Disease And Emotional Issues

Healing emotional baggage is the mantra to live healthy and happy life. The longer the emotional baggage is piled up, the severe the disease becomes. Diseases are the wake-up call for us to realize that enough is enough. Shed your emotional baggage. It is very important to know what emotional blockages are causing what disease. You can do aura scan or Byosen scan or any scanning technique you know to find out which chakra is out of balance and analyze the emotional blockage related to the chakra. Start healing your issues with Divine light of Reiki. Reiki helps and treats on physical, mental and emotional level. Healing with reiki helps resolve some unresolved long pending issues. Reiki clears long-piled-up blockages and clears long built-up toxins from all levels- Emotional, Physical and Mental.

The front side of our body represents to social life, the part of you that you share with the world. Also represents love, happiness, sadness, desire and care.

The back side of our body represents private life. The part of you that is hidden from world. This side becomes a storeroom where all your hidden emotions accumulate. Unexpressed emotions piling up. It means negativity accumulating along your spine and legs.

The left side of the body represents feminine side.

The right side of the body represents masculine side.

Below is a chart that will help analyze your body, disease and emotional blockages associated. Start giving divine Reiki energy to your emotional blockages to get rid of long accumulated negativity piled up in your body.

Body/Disease	Emotional Cause

Abdominal problems	Stopping some process, Fear
Abuse	Inadequacy, Lack of self-love
Aching	Craving for love
Acne	Self-dislike
Addiction	Not facing fear, Lack of self-love
Alcoholism	Self-rejection, Guilt
Allergies	Blockage in intestine/stomach, Unable to digest issues
Alzheimer	Denial to see and accept the world as it is
Anorexia	Fear of rejection

Ankle problem	Inflexibility, Inability to accept the joys of life, Need to change direction
Anxiety	Unresolved fear of past experience
Arm problem	Capacity to hold life experiences; Right- Regret Left-Helplessness
Arthritis	Inflexibility, Feel unloved
Asthma	Stifled emotions, Past lives fears acknowledged in this life
Athlete's foot	Unable to move forward with ease

Back	Lack of support, Money issues, Unloved, Stored anger
Baldness	Tension
Bladder	Fear of letting go
Blood Pressure	Blockages in freedom, Unsolved emotional problems
Blood problem	Lack of joy
Bones	Past lives and Memories
Breast(Left)	Lack of nurture
Breast(Right)	Resistance is sharing love, Overprotection
Bronchitis	Helplessness caused by the feeling of not able to change

Burns	situation Suppressed inner anger
Calves	Moving forward and avoiding past issues
Cancer	Unresolved deep hurt
Cavity	Unable to accept new concepts
Chest	Relationship issues, Feel worthless, low self-esteem
Chronic Disease	Feel unsafe, Unable to change
Cold	Mental Confusion
Cold hands and feet	Lack of self-trust
Cold & flu	It symbolizes

	cleansing
Colon	Not accepting changes for emotional reasons
Coma	Escaping from situation or people
Constipation	Hanging on to old beliefs
Cramps/Stiffness	Unable to adjust to natural changes in life
Depression	Feel unloved-unwanted, Unrevealed anger
Digestive problem	Suppressed anger. Unable to accept certain things
Dizziness	Scattered thoughts

Ear	Denial to hear
Elbow	Inflexibility, Unable to accept new changes
Eyes	How we see the world. Not seeing things clearly knowingly or unknowingly. Not wanting to open eyes, Fear of today
Eyes (Nearsighted)	They tend to live for today; no future plan, Fear of the future
Eyes (Far-sighted)	They keep planning future that leads their thoughts to confusions
Flabs	Sadness, Holding other's or your own

Feet	emotion in your body Related to security and survival. Have you taken wrong direction in life?
Fever	Anger
Flu	Body indicating you to slow down
Fibroids	Confusion about being loved, Holding on to pain for long
Frigidity	Denial of joy. Bad feelings towards sexual pleasures
Gas	Indigestible ideas
Gum problem	Not sticking to decision, Unable to make decision
Hands	Holding on or letting

go

Headache/Hitting your head	It is a wakeup call to pay attention to the things you have been ignoring. Do not ignore your intuitions.
Head(back side) Neck base	Guilt, Unable to forgive yourself, You believe you have some mistake, harsh behavior inflicted by others or yourself
Hearing problem	Not wanting to hear what is going on around you
Heart problem	Not listening/ignoring our feelings
Heart attack	Favoring money or status, ignoring joys of life, lack of love
Hips	General support-

	feeling of lack of support, Fear to take a step further related to big issues
Insomnia	Fear/guilt
Joints	Inflexibility, Stubbornness regarding certain situations and your attachment to it
Kidney	Anger- Holding on to anger
Kidney Stone	Unresolved anger
Knees	Holding on to past anger, feel unsupported Inside knee- Job, Friend/Social issues.
Legs	Fear of change, fear of future, family or

	parental issues
Lungs/Heart	Not sharing love
Migraine	Unreleased anger, Sexual fear, Unreleased anger
Mouth	Unable to speak-up, Suppressed thoughts
Muscles	Inability to move on
Nail biting	Questioning your worth
Neck	Stubborn, Stiff, Denial to see other's point of view
Nerves	Sensitivity towards certain issues that are not acknowledged in the

	conscious mind
Numbness	Going dead mentally. Giving up
Osteoporosis	Feeling lack of support
Ovaries	Sensitive past issues(creativity), Guilt
Over-weight	Carrying past lives burden, Insecurity, Craving for love
Paralysis	Helplessness
Pimples	Anger outburst
Pneumonia	Giving up
PMS	Rejection of feminine problems

Ringworms	Allowing others to affect you
Sciatica	Financial problems
Sinus	Confusion, Irritation towards one person
Slipped disc	Lack of support
Skin	Anxiety
Snoring	Unable to get rid of old ideas
Stomach	Unable to digest certain issues
Stroke	Giving up on life
Stuttering	Insecurity
Swelling	Unshed tears

Teeth	Past life pain coming out to be released, indecisiveness
Throat	Unable to speak up for self, Swollen anger
Thumb	Always worrying
Thyroid	Feel humiliated, Lack of freedom
Ulcers	Feel unfulfilled
Urinal problem	Anger towards opposite sex
Varicose veins	Feel over-burdened, not liking the present situation
Vomiting	Rejection of new ideas

Blessed Stones

We all know the concept of Lucky Charms/Lucky mascots. It is believed to bring good luck. It can be carried around, worn or can be placed anywhere in your home or work place. These lucky charms doesn't have to be any Feng-sui or religious based thing. When you see something that attracts you, appeals to you or makes you all excited than you will know this is IT.

I have my own way of making my lucky charm. I call it 'Blessed Stone'. All you need is a stone, your creativity and reiki. You can decorate the stone the way you want. Paint it, design it or stick stickers. You can use this 'Blessed Stone' for various purpose.

- As Reiki Bank
- As your personalized stone

- As a gift to your students and clients
- Gift to loved ones

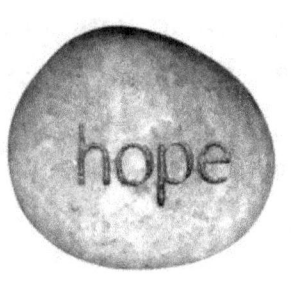

Here is what you need to do.
- Find a stone that fits in palm. Feel it, see if it feels right. Your intuition will guide you. If the stone is white, you can be more creative with it.
- Wash the stone. Keep it plain or paint it with the color of your choice.

Decorate it with designs or dots, whatever you want.
- You can personalize the stone by writing name or message on it. I have made a stone with my name written on it. Have

made for kids with their own name personalized on the stone.
- Once the stone is ready, Draw reiki symbols over it and bless the stone with reiki energy. Put in your intention along with reiki energy. Your 'Blessed Stone' is ready.
- Carry this 'Blessed Stone' with you or place it at your sacred place.

My 'Blessed Stone' is my Reiki Bank. Whenever I feel drained, stuck or in a fix I take out my 'Blessed Stone' and hold it in my palms to get revived. I withdraw reiki from my 'Blessed Stone' especially when I am unwell. You can deposit reiki energy to this 'Blessed Stone' the same way you deposit reiki to Reiki Bank.

You can personalize this 'Blessed Stone' by writing your family or friend's name and infuse it with reiki with the intention that's meant for them. Ask them to carry the stone with them as their lucky charm.

You can even personalize this 'Blessed Stone' for your students and give them as a gift. Personalize it for your client and infuse with reiki with the intention to heal them. Ask them to use this 'Blessed Stone' as a Reiki Bank or as a lucky charm.

Instead of stones, you can use shells too for this same purpose. Be creative and use lots of reiki. That's it □

Chapter 12: Reiki For Self-Healing

As touched on previously, Reiki for self-treatments is highly beneficial and important for a Reiki practitioner. Once you have received your attunements, your connection to Reiki and the universe will be stronger. One of the best ways to foster that connection is practice. You are your best practice subject. Also as a practitioner, you will be working closely with others, and while you cannot take on their energetic burdens, working with clients who are injured or have emotional traumas can be heavy work. Using Reiki on yourself will help keep your energy and body in the best condition.

There is always more to learn when it comes to Reiki and energy. After completing your course, keep yourself open to learning more and trying new things. Using yourself for practice allows you to try out new things if you aren't yet comfortable with trying them on a client.

Keep practicing on yourself to build your confidence.

When you first receive your attunements and are starting on your healing journey with Reiki, it is best to focus on yourself. Healing your own imbalances with Reiki will better prepare you for working with clients. It could also very well change your entire life and help you discover more about yourself and your own path.

Many of the greatest healers have struggled with emotional, physical, or spiritual traumas or burdens. Reiki is almost unique in the sense that you can use it on yourself. It isn't selfish to take the time and focus to work on what you need before taking Reiki to the next step of working with others.

Every session will feel different, this includes sessions you perform on yourself. Give yourself some realistic expectations about your own comfort and practice with Reiki energy. It will get stronger and feel more natural the more you practice.

In some instances where practitioners focus only on healing others and not using Reiki on themselves, they may be quite effective in the healing room, but their lives outside of their healing space are quite different. In their personal lives, they might struggle with low vibrations, not live by the five Reiki principles, or struggle in other areas of their lives.

To be the highest version of yourself and the best Reiki practitioner, Reiki should be a lifestyle. It should be a part of you and your every day's tasks and actions. Not just a service you provide for others.

The greatest benefit you can provide others is by healing and balancing yourself. That energy will them affect them even if they are in close proximity to you, not just from receiving a Reiki session. The world can benefit simply from your presence when you reach that naturally balanced state.

The more your energy changes and balances, the more your vibration and frequency change, the greater you can affect your environment, draw to you what you most want in life, and impact the people that are closest to you. With Reiki, sometimes balance and peace are the greatest rewards, because once you are balanced and at peace, you can truly accomplish anything.

Self-imposed barriers are removed, limitations get lifted, you can see the bigger picture and have a clarity of mind that allows you to progress how and where you want to. Releasing the belief that we aren't good enough, or that we can't make money following our passions, or that we have to work hard for what we want is entirely liberating. Reiki can provide that liberation and allow you to actually start living how you want!

With Reiki, you can also learn a lot about yourself and come to terms with a lot of things you deal with day to day. Reiki is there for you and can be a huge support. If you're tired, give yourself a boost with

Reiki. If you feel down or sad, lift your spirits with a little Reiki. The uses are infinite, especially for yourself.

Reiki will help your body-mind get to the source of any imbalance in your body and that will only benefit you and your life. Performing Reiki on yourself every day will help you recharge your body and your own energy. The body is a machine. Like all machines, it requires maintenance, care, and alterations. Reiki is a natural source of energy to provide the body with all the maintenance and care it needs!

A poorly maintained car gets rust, parts break, it starts to make strange sounds, doesn't drive straight, and little things start to pile up until it is no longer usable. Your body and energy are the same! Every day actions such as driving, sitting at a desk all day, running, construction work, yard work, things that seem mundane cause wear and tear. So does fatigue, emotional stress, domestic tension, anger outbursts, and other emotional build-ups.

Rather than the body starting to make strange sounds and no longer being able to drive straight, we develop injuries, illnesses, even diseases. Some are physical, some are emotional, and some are mental. Daily Reiki treatments for yourself are the maintenance to keep these at bay. Reiki is your daily oil change, alignment, filled gas tank, filled washer fluid, brake line check, light check, and full-body car wash in one!

Benefits of Daily Self-Treatments

Reiki self-treatments provide you with more than just a way to practice and hone your skills as a practitioner. There are physical, mental, and spiritual benefits of Reiki that you can provide yourself with every day!

Benefits of Reiki:

Reiki will provide you with relaxation

Reiki brings you mental clarity

Reiki can give you an energy boost

Reiki calms you

Reiki gives you insight into solving problems

Reiki relieves physical and emotional pain

Reiki promotes and accelerates the natural healing process

Reiki prevents and slows the progress of disease and illness

Reiki purifies and detoxifies the physical and energetic body

Reiki fixes energy blocks

Reiki releases emotional blocks

Reiki changes the vibrational frequency of the body

Reiki helps promote positivity and break negative habits and behaviors

These are just a few of the benefits that practitioners feel daily when they give themselves treatments. Reiki benefits don't have to be huge an immediately noticeable. Sometimes, they are more subtle. While it is great to set some time aside every day to perform a full Reiki session for yourself, sometimes life gets in the way and you have to improvise.

Maybe you are getting a headache at work, place your hand on your head and do a quick five-minute session for yourself. Maybe you need a little extra boost to get yourself out of bed in the morning, place your hands on your stomach and give yourself a little Reiki to help get up and get moving.

Self-Treatment can be used for more targeted benefits, like a headache or energy boost. The Bodymind knows what needs to be addressed with Reiki if you are experiencing a specific symptom, but that five or ten-minute quick session can target your symptom quickly and allow you to get on with your day.

How to Perform a Self-Treatment

Many new Reiki practitioners have this concern that they aren't 'doing it right.' Energy work is subjective, much like art. There isn't necessarily a right or wrong way to perform a session on yourself. Most likely, you will start with a routine in the beginning and then as you get more comfortable, start to modify or change that routine as needed.

Even though as a Reiki practitioner, you don't target a specific symptom, sometimes starting a session with your hands over a painful or afflicted area can benefit the session. Some practitioners will start on a painful area of themselves and then continue with the remaining hand positions as normal.

A common question with new students is 'If Reiki goes where it is needed, why are there hand positions?' Generally, the hand positions are an effort to limit conscious resistance on the practitioner or client's part. This is especially true when working with clients as they often like to feel the whole body being worked on with physical touch. However, when working on yourself, you don't have to use hand positions if you feel comfortable enough performing Reiki without them.

Even in personal use though, placing the hands over a specifically painful area can create a conscious feeling of relief just by having a physical focus on the painful area. Hand positions can also be a part of the treatment process and determining where there are energy blocks or areas that need attention. You may sometimes notice yourself avoiding certain hand positions or positioning your hands over certain areas of your body.

If this is the case, going back to performing a full-body self-treatment or adding additional hand positions might be beneficial. You may avoid an area subconsciously for many reasons, and if you find that to be the case, understanding why you are avoiding that area may help you in your self-healing.

In the beginning, it is especially helpful to follow a routine and the suggested hand positions. This will also help you to learn what positions are used during treatment on a client as many are similar, or placed similarly on the body. However, once you are familiar with the recommended positions, your intuition can guide you as to what positions work best for you.

During a self-treatment, get comfortable. Play some relaxing music, light a few candles and dim the lights. Burn some incense or diffuse and essential oil. Try to pick a place that won't be disturbed during your self-treatment. This will ensure the highest vibration of work.

Try to set aside between 30 and 45 minutes a day to perform a self-treatment of Reiki on yourself. This should become part of your daily routine and lifestyle. To really live the Reiki life and be a strong, practiced practitioner, giving yourself the proper time to heal and soak up Reiki energy is important.

There is no right or wrong time to perform a session. If you'd rather wake up and do a session that is great. If you'd prefer to perform a session at night or take a break in the middle of the day, any option works. You will need to decide which time is best for you and your lifestyle and schedule.

That being said, a self-treatment doesn't have to be performed at the same time every day. Work it in where you can.

As you perform the hand positions on yourself, each position should be held between 3 and 5 minutes. You may find yourself needing to spend more or less time on specific areas. Allow your intuition to guide you.

Generally speaking, a little Reiki is better than no Reiki. If there are days that you don't have time for a 30 or 45-minute self-treatment, do what you can. It is said that shortening the time you hold hand positions is better than skipping hand positions all together if you are strapped for time.

Another option if you don't have a lot of time is doing smaller sessions on yourself when you can, 5 to 15 minutes throughout the day. It is worth noting, that these should be balanced out with full-body self-treatments when you can do them, but it is still better to perform a smaller session on yourself than none at all.

At the beginning of every self-Reiki session, try setting an intention for yourself. Your intention should be to heal yourself on all levels and balance yourself on all levels. Use your breath in your self-treatments. With every inhale, visualize yourself drawing Reiki into your body-mind. As you exhale, imagine yourself releasing energy that no longer serves your highest health and good.

Be present in your sessions. Teach yourself how to focus on the Reiki and not have your mind wandering. This is important for self-sessions but also sessions with clients. There is nothing more disheartening for a client to be on the table and feel like their practitioner is thinking about anything but them!

Being present is incredibly important during a Reiki session. This is called conscious touch, thinking of your client, even if that client is you during a self-treatment. If your mind is wandering to what you are going to be making for dinner later that night, or who you are hanging out with this weekend, that can impede the energy flow.

It may seem unrealistic, but clients can and do feel and pick up on those absent-minded feelings from their practitioner. Working on yourself is a great way to practice presence and mindfulness while treating yourself and others. Meditation is another great method for practicing mindfulness.

After your self-treatment is completed, make sure to drink a glass of cold water. Keep yourself hydrated in between Reiki sessions. Make sure to properly close your session and the energetic flow with a deep breath and intend that the Reiki session is complete. Make sure to thank your own body, Reiki energies, and any other forces you give thanks to at the end of a session.

At the end of your session, you can say an affirmation to affirm that you have received the healing and balance you need from your Reiki session. Many Reiki practitioners also like to touch each other their seven main chakras at the end of a Reiki session.

Some common feelings that arise after a session can include lightheadedness, fatigue, or just lethargy. Give yourself a little time to recover if you need to. Practicing a grounding exercise, or just slowly ease back into activity.

If you fall asleep during a self-treatment, the next treatment you perform on yourself, pick up at the last hand position you remember leaving off at before falling asleep.

It is not uncommon to see visions, colors, or get specific feelings or ideas while you are giving yourself a Reiki session. If you'd like, keep a journal or notebook nearby to record what you see and feel. Then you can take the time to understand what they meant to you.

Self-Treatment Hand Positions

The following self-treatment hand positions are a guideline for how to perform the treatment. Not every self-treatment has to be long or ceremonious. You can also use whatever hand positions feel right for yourself.

The self-treatment hand positions are designed for ease and comfort while performing a session on yourself. Generally sitting down is the best way to go. However, lying down is sometimes more comfortable. Lying down does run the risk of you falling asleep in some instances. If you are not ready to go to bed, sitting might be the best option for performing self-treatments.

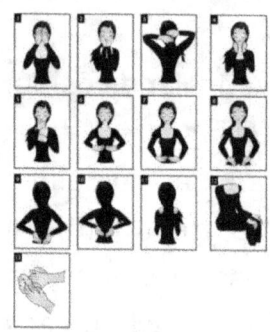

Many practitioners will wait until they are going to bed to perform a self-treatment though because it assists in their ability to get to sleep. If you are lying down, some of the hand positions may need to be modified.

Consistent Self-Treatments

Over time, you might come to find that your commitment to performing Reiki treatments on yourself begins to dwindle. This is common with practitioners, but also unfortunate. In order to provide an effective healing service to others, or to the entire world, you need to be balanced in yourself. Reiki isn't just a tool for healing and balancing. Reiki has the amazing ability to increase awareness and clarity. These benefits are highly important when practicing Reiki as a service for clients.

Throughout our lives we grow, we change, and we heal our past, present, and future. Without properly balancing ourselves we can shift back into unhealthy habits, negative thinking, and lost sight of what it is that we wanted to accomplish by starting down the Reiki path.

It is possible for healing and change to occur spontaneously, however, it is more likely that it needs to be stimulated or encouraged. Using Reiki every day to treat yourself will continue to encourage growth and change in your life rather than regression.

Our current society idealizes immediate gratification. People don't want something if they can't see immediate results or feel better immediately, pain-free instantly. This mentality has contributed to many issues including obesity and opioid addiction. There is no magic fix or cure-all that will instantly take the pain away and make the world better. It is unfortunate, but true healing and balance and growth take time!

If you feel like you are wasting your time by performing self-treatments, or like too much time has passed without benefit, remember that it does take time. Brushing your teeth and flossing is to maintain dental health and prevent cavities. You still do it every day, even though you don't see that plaque being scrubbed from your teeth.

In the same way, Reiki should be worked into your daily routine. Even if you don't feel or see immediate results, it is the long term benefit and the continued care and balance that you want to maintain.

Saying you don't have time or energy to perform a daily Reiki session is just another way to limit and restrict yourself with society imposed beliefs. Your time is your own. Your health is your priority, and

Reiki is a tool that can momentously change your health.

If Reiki is an interest of yours and you want to study it and learn how to use it and heal others, remember that the most important starting point is in healing yourself. Choose to follow a more positive, balanced, aware lifestyle that will benefit yourself, your environment, and those around you by treating yourself with Reiki daily.

Chapter 13: How Reiki Increase Your Energy, Reduce Stress, Depression And Improve Your Health

Reiki is a Japanese approach that also encourages healing for stress reduction and relaxation. It is administered by the setting of hands and is easy for anyone to learn.
Reiki Is In Your Hands As A Health Toolbox. Reiki is a deep instrument for self-care use. Indeed, most Reiki practitioners who studied Reiki healing practice on a daily basis some sort of Self-Reiki. One lovely element of Reiki is that you have the understanding and use it for life once you take a Reiki class. It's always in your hands for you, a wellness toolbox. An individual may often have been searching for Reiki for healing advantages. Your doctor or medical provider may have learned about it. You might have heard excellent friends or family outcomes. Or in the media, like

on the Dr. Oz show, you may have heard about it.

Reiki Works!

In recent decades, Reiki has achieved popularity because—it operates! People who have been fortunate enough to receive a Reiki session or series of Reiki sessions often want to take a Reiki One or First Degree Reiki class. After taking Reiki 1, you've got a starting set of instruments you can use in self-care anytime, anywhere. A Calming, lasting benefit can be provided by five minutes of Reiki a day. Reiki calms you down and centers you like meditation. Also, Reiki energizes and also offers clarity of mind. This is because both providing relaxation and strengthening and assisting the power pathways of your body to work optimally work energetically.

Reiki for Self Care: Practical, Everyday Applications

Some of Self-Reiki's practical applications include: getting ready for the day, using Reiki to calm down in traffic, ten minutes of Reiki to add calm before going to bed, five minutes before your presentation, five minutes of Reiki to get you to calm down and help others, and an endless array of situations. You can use Reiki with your animals and friends to prepare meals, gardening as well. But keep in mind that self-care is important to keep you at your best, so you can do wonders a few minutes of self-reiki a day.

Reiki Healing for Personal Growth, Relaxation, Stress Reduction, Comfort, and Clarity

You understand how strong and deep this lovely modality can be if you've taken a Reiki Level I course. It is a toolbox, literally in your hands, to reduce stress, convenience, and clarity. And each consecutive Reiki level brings another level of depth with it.

How Reiki can increase productivity

Creativity comes in many ways, whether it is music making, yard art forging, or even finding an incredible answer to a worldly issue. And Reiki has the authority to fuel your creativity into realms that you might never have believed possible. Here's how and why you can increase your creativity with Reiki. Reiki can boost your productivity by minimizing stress and over-sized ego Stress and ego are like two good friends, often hand in hand galloping. The ego's self-centered, hyperactive, compulsive nature can in fact generate stress in some instances. Stress can also cause the need for control in other cases, calling the ego into full gear. One of the biggest advantages of Reiki can be a fast decrease in stress concentrations that can simultaneously deflate an overbearing ego. You will automatically gain access to the greater mind's creative arena once you are free to look at other good convictions and choices.

Helps Clears Energetic Blocks

The only thing that can block the free flow of creativity are not ego and stress. Another culprit is energetic blocks. The capacity of Reiki to clear these vigorous blocks gives you fresh inspiration and opens the possibility that it wants to flow freely, piercing your imagination and producing thoughts. Releasing these blocks can also provide access to your shadow self or greater nature, improving your ability to know at all levels.

How Reiki Can Boost Your Creativity

Creativity comes in many ways, whether it is music making, yard art forging, or even finding an incredible answer to a worldly issue. And Reiki has the authority to fuel your creativity into realms that you might never have believed possible. Here's how and why you can increase your creativity with Reiki. Reiki your bed for a better night's sleep. Reiki your clothes and jewelry so that as you wear them, they maintain you calm and focused all day. Reiki your electronics so that when your computer runs slowly or you see something that would normally irritate you on social media, you don't get stressed out.

Reiki your Medications

You can even use your Reiki medicines to make them even more healing and nutritious for you. You can use Reiki any item to create it healthier and softer to use. Make your life as you use Reiki on today's everyday objects and whenever they need a "tune-up."

Chapter 14: Positions For The Application

Head Area
First Head Position
a) Physical body
Works on any problem with the eyes, vision, colors, clarity (photophobia), glaucoma, cataracts, injuries, irritations, and conjunctivitis
Nose problems, allergic rhinitis, spongy meat, septum deviation, and respiratory congestion
Problems with the jaws, jaw, gums, teeth, pH of the mucous membranes, and mouth
Bone cavity problems (sinusitis)
Headache, migraine, effusions, allergy, colds, and asthma
It balances the pituitary gland, which is also called the pituitary gland. This is located in the center of the skull on the Turkish chair. It is considered the main gland since it has as its function is the balance of the whole body system and "tells" the other glands what they should

do. The pituitary gland is the master gland of the endocrine system. It influences growth, sexual development, fatigue, gravity, lactation, metabolism, the dosage of sugar and minerals in the blood, fluid retention, and energy levels.

It balances the pineal gland, which is also called the epiphysis; that gland is located at the base of the skull base. It is small, the size of a pea, and responds to the levels of light that the eyes perceive, thanks to the secretion of the hormone melatonin. It has an important role in the mood. Many refer to that gland as the third eye, the gland of intuition, or paranormality.

b) Emotional body

Reduce stress

Relieves anxiety

Provides relaxation, even at the neurological level

c) Mental body

Relieves and reduces mental confusion and generates balance and clarity of thoughts and ideas

Allows increasing the capacity of concentration and centralization of the individual

d) Spiritual body

It balances the sixth chakra.

It lets us penetrate our inner selves to be in touch with our own wisdom.

It opens us to higher energies.

It allows you to lose the feeling of duality and achieve the feeling of uniqueness with the divine laws.

It expands and helps purify consciousness.

It benefits the level of spiritual devotion, favoring meditation, and the state of concentration.

Second Head Position

a) Physical body

It works directly with the brain, balancing the right and left sides and encouraging production, creativity, thoughts, and memory.

It balances the pituitary and pineal glands.

It works on cerebral dysrhythmia, seizures, and aneurysms.

It quickly relieves headaches and migraines.

It assists in the recovery of people who are drugged or intoxicated.

b) Emotional body

Reduce worries, hysteria, and stress

It helps relieve depression, anguish, and fears (all pathological states of panic).

Promotes relaxation

It balances the person in cases where emotion or reasoning predominates.

c) Mental body

Works on mental illnesses (psychosis, neurosis, schizophrenia)

Develops clarity of thoughts, induces serenity, and stimulates the speed of responses

Stimulates a clearer vision of life and problems

d) Spiritual body

Increases the ability to receive higher energies

Expands awareness and interaction with cosmic wisdom (Akashic record)

Promotes the memory of dreams and previous lives (insights)

Third Head Position

a)   Physical body

Harmonizes the functioning of the pituitary gland or pituitary gland

Works with the marrow and the brain

Covers the base of the brain, harmonizing the functions performed by the cerebellum, which is located in the back of the cranial cavity

Decreases neck tension and relaxes the upper part of the cervical vertebrae

Regulates sleep, helps you sleep due to lack of sleep, and helps you wake up due to excessive sleepiness

The occipital lobe that is located in the back of the brain works, where the vision centers are located

Regulates weight and hunger

Acts on problems related to speech and stuttering

Relieves headaches at the base of the skull

Works with people who are in a state of shock by accident, in a coma, or fainting

Works on any vice, reducing the compulsion

Works on coordination and balance (labyrinthitis)

b) Emotional body

It develops the well-being and promotes relaxing and calm thoughts.

It reduces stress, depression, irritations, worries, fears, and traumas.

c) Mental body

Clarity of expression of thought and ideas

Promotes serenity, creativity, and productivity

d) Spiritual body

Works on the sixth chakra (Ajna) on its back.

Expands the reception of higher energies

Promotes the memory of dreams and past lives

Opening of the third eye and developing the instincts (eyes and inner ears) and paranormality (ability to enter an altered state of consciousness, astral projection, clairvoyance, clairaudience, telepathy, psychography, etc.).

Fourth Head Position

a) Physical body

It works with metabolism, thyroid, and parathyroid glands. The thyroid gland is located in the lower third of the neck, in front of the trachea. It regulates metabolism and growth. The parathyroid glands consist of four tiny corpuscles linked to the thyroid. They control calcium metabolism, contributing to the control of muscle tone.

It works on the jaws, jaws, tonsils, throat, and pharynx.

It works on the salivary glands.

It works on the lymphatic drainage and upper cervical nodes.

It balances blood pressure (high and low).

The throat is a center of expression, creativity, and communication.

b) Emotional body

Works to neutralize feelings such as anger, hostility, resentment, nervousness, and fears of failure

Develops self-esteem and self-confidence

c) Mental body

It develops calm, relaxation, decreased critical sense, well-being, clarity, mental stability, tranquility, and pleasure to live.

d) Spiritual body

It works on the fifth chakra (laryngeal or Vishuda).

It helps to keep in tune with spirituality in a more creative and sincere way.

Front Area

First Position Forward

a) Physical body

It works with the heart, circulation, veins, and arteries that leave the heart.

It harmonizes the lungs in the upper part and the functions of the bronchi.

It covers part of the trachea.

It helps in lymphatic drainage.

It balances the thymus that, in childhood, performs important endocrine and immunological functions. Although it is reduced in the adult, its influence on the organism is still felt, as regards immunology.

Conclusion

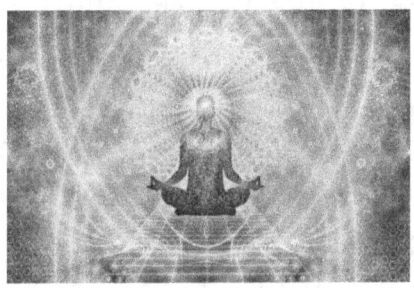

Now that you have completed this part of the series, the next step to take is to find a Reiki Master or practitioner. If you have not already done so, look for a practitioner that you resonate with so you can begin your Reiki Level I course. Make sure to find a practitioner who you feel comfortable with and one that you resonate with.

As you search for a Reiki Master, start making mediation practices a regular part of your daily routine. This is going to be the first step in clearing yourself and releasing unwanted energies so that when you receive your Reiki attunement ceremony, you'll be more open and aligned to those energies. If you can, make small shifts in your diet and lifestyle to help foster open energetic channels as you continue down this path of personal healing and personal empowerment.

Since the path you have chosen to walk is going to create shifts in your body, mind, spirit, and your physical environment, begin keeping a journal or notebook of your experiences. This is going to help you track the subtle shifts and changes, and also give you a way to reflect back on your progress.

www.ingramcontent.com/pod-product-compliance
Lightning Source LLC
Chambersburg PA
CBHW072013070526
44583CB00015B/1455